Brain

51 Powerful Ways to Improve Brain Power, Enhance Memory, Intelligence and Concentration

NATURALLY!

New and Improved – 2nd Edition

Shining Universe Energy Books

Table of Contents –

Introduction

We want to thank you and congratulate you for buying our book, "Brain: 51 Powerful Ways to Improve Brain Power, Enhance Memory, Intelligence and Concentration NATURALLY!"

This book contains proven steps and strategies on how to improve brain power, open up areas of the brain and enhance memory, intelligence and concentration.

Have you ever wondered why human beings are the most powerful creatures on this planet? It is not the size of the body or the strength of the muscles but the presence of an extremely sophisticated brain that has allowed us to master this planet.

Do you know that though the structure or the anatomy of the brain is identical in all human beings, only a few, perhaps less than 5% are able to use it to the full potential by developing it? The other 95% live out their lives without harnessing the full potential of the brain and sadly majority of them do not even know that they can enhance their brain power through simple techniques and considerably improve the overall quality of their lives.

This book will attempt to explain in detail about the brain, how it functions, the difference between a genius and an ordinary brain and finally we will reveal the secrets of how to improve your brain power through extremely well-researched 51 powerful ways, NATURALLY!

Besides this, we have also included 14 fabulous brain exercises that will help you transform your brain, sharpen your memory, concentration and focus thus helping you lead a better life.

Because this is a brand new edition, we have improved the book with an additional 21 brand new ways to improve the brain, focusing on how to enhance brain development throughout the stages of childhood.

Thank you again for getting this book. We really hope you will like it and benefit immensely.

Also included along with this book are your BONUS GIFTS – 5 Additional High Quality Books – Only for you!

You can get them at the end of this book.

Chapter 1: The Brain - Its Importance and Potential

The brain is the human body's most complex organ. It initiates body movement, it controls behavior, it interprets the five senses, and – most importantly – it is the pinnacle of intelligence. Immersed in protective fluid and nestled in its bony shell, the approximately three-pound brain is the origin of what defines humanity's qualities. Since the brain is the body's most important organ, you can say that it is the human body's crown jewel.

Philosophers and scientists, for centuries, have been enthralled by the brain and, until recently, they saw the brain as nearly inscrutable. Nowadays, the brain is just starting to reveal its secrets. In the past 10 years, scientists have unlocked some of the brain's mysteries. We have learned about it more today than in the prior centuries due to the fast pace of modern research in behavioral and neurological science. We have also formulated new research techniques.

The U.S. Congress thus named the 1990s as the 'Decade of the Brain.' At the forefront of the research efforts is the NINDS (National Institute of Neurological Disorders and Stroke), which supports and conducts scientific research in the United States and all over the world.

The Brain's Importance

Science has already established the fact that the brain is the body's command center. Everything you say, do, and think about involves the power and function of the brain.

This central organ can be broken down into two different regions or hemispheres (left and right), each of which performs different functions including balance, speech, and movement. Any damage to a particular region of the brain can affect the function it controls. That would lead to symptoms like difficulty speaking, loss of concentration, or loss of movement.

The brain's left hemisphere controls the sensory and motor functions of the right side of the human body. It is also in charge of logical and scientific functions like understanding spoken and written language, reasoning, and number skills. The brain's right hemisphere controls the left side of the body's sensory and motor functions. The brain's right side takes care of artistic functions like insight, art awareness, and music.

Improved Brain Power: How it Affects the Body

Enhanced brain power can help you in all aspects of your life. A brain that is constantly conditioned can help improve your body's overall functions. A constantly conditioned and healthy brain can help you overcome negative emotions and stress. Thus, it is important that you eat right, indulge in physical exercise, and do some mental exercises as well. These will help boost brainpower and sharpen the mind. You will learn more about how to improve your brain power in the later chapters.

Enhancing your brain power can also prevent or slow the progress of degenerative nervous system conditions like peripheral neuropathies, Huntington's disease, Alzheimer's disease, or Parkinson's disease, among other neurological-related conditions. This book, however, will center more on improving your brain's general functions rather than these specific conditions.

Brain Power Boost at any Age

A strong memory depends on the brain's vitality and health. Whether you're a working professional wanting to stay sharp and ahead of your game or a senior citizen who wants to enhance and preserve your gray matter as you grow older, there are many things you can do to improve your mental performance and memory.

The age-old adage "you can't teach an old dog new tricks" does not apply to the human brain. Even in old age, the human brain has the astounding ability to change and adapt. It is known as neuroplasticity. Your brain, with the proper stimulation, can alter existing connections, form new neural pathways, and react and adapt in constantly changing ways.

It is true that the brain can greatly reshape itself when it concerns memory and learning. You can enhance neuroplasticity and increase your natural power to learn new info, increase and improve your cognitive abilities, and – at any age – improve your memory.

Chapter 2: Basics of the Brain

Just like any bodily organ, the brain has different parts that work together. Each part has its unique abilities and functions. The brain is divided into three fundamental units: forebrain, midbrain, and hindbrain. These units are the most essential building blocks for the rest of the brain, and all three are fully formed by six weeks' gestation. Each unit in turn contains a number of smaller sections essential for optimal brain functioning.

The forebrain is the human brain's most highly-developed section; it is also the largest part of the organ. It consists of the cerebrum and the sub-structures beneath it. The forebrain is responsible for regulating many of the basic functions needed for a healthy life, such as eating, drinking, sleeping, and reproduction. It also is the part of the brain that enables humans to show their emotions.

The midbrain, which is the brainstem's uppermost part, controls several reflex actions and is an integral part of the circuit that helps control certain voluntary movements as well as eye movements. The hindbrain includes the spinal cord's upper part, the cerebellum (a wrinkled tissue ball), and the brain stem. The hindbrain takes care of vital bodily functions like heart rate and respiration. The cerebellum, which coordinates movement, is in charge of any learned routine movements and hearing. Along with the forebrain, it plays important roles in regulating sleep cycles and body temperatures.

Most of the signals from the brain to the body (and vice-versa) will traverse on their way from and to the brain in somewhat opposing or polarized directions. It means that the brain's right hemisphere mainly controls the body's left side and the left hemisphere takes care of the right side. If a particular side of the brain is impaired, the body's opposite side is affected instead. An example would be a stroke on the brain's right side, which can leave the left leg and left arm paralyzed.

How Thoughts are Created

Each cerebral hemisphere has lobes (sections), each of which has various functions. The 2 frontal lobes are located directly behind the forehead. When you think about the future, use reasoned arguments, or plan a schedule, the two lobes are working. The frontal lobes function as short-term memory storage sites, enabling an idea to be kept in the mind. Other ideas to be considered and remembered for the time being are stored here as well. Additionally, the frontal lobe is the part of the brain largely responsible for foreseeing future consequences of actions we might take today. It is what enables humans to weigh risk versus reward and plan our actions accordingly. Finally, this lobe modifies our emotional reactions in order to fit the norms and customs of the society and culture we feel familiar with, lessening the chances of us even desiring to do something that the general public would view negatively.

The rearmost portion of each lobe functions as a motor-function control area that manages the body's voluntary movement. Near the left frontal lobe is known as the *Broca's area*, which enables thoughts to come out as spoken words. This part of the brain was named after Pierre Paul Broca, a French physician who discovered its function in his research efforts in the year 1861. Broca's area is so important to speech and communication in general that damage to it significantly impairs natural hand motions, making sign languages and even nonverbal communications a significant challenge.

The parietal lobes, which are two sections behind the frontal lobes, are responsible for culinary enjoyment – they are the part that tells you the food's texture, aroma, and taste. The primary sensory areas, which are behind the motor areas and are the forward parts of the parietal lobes, receive information on touch, taste, movement, and temperature from the rest of the body. Arithmetic and reading are also considered the parietal lobes' responsibility.

The occipital lobes, which are located at the rear of the brain, process images from the eyes and connect that information with memory-stored images. Damage to these lobes may lead to blindness, and abnormalities within the lobes is responsible for between five and ten percent of all epilepsy cases.

Lastly, the temporal lobes lie in front of the visual areas and rest under the frontal and parietal lobes. They are responsible as you appreciate rock music or symphonies. On top of each temporal lobe is an area that manages the information gathered using the ears. Each temporal lobe underside is responsible for retrieving and forming memories, including the ones linked to music. The temporal lobe is what enables us to recognize and remember the faces and voices of those we interact with, as well as working in tandem with Broca's area to enable us to comprehend speech. Other parts of the temporal lobe seem to integrate sensations and memories of sound, taste, touch, and sight.

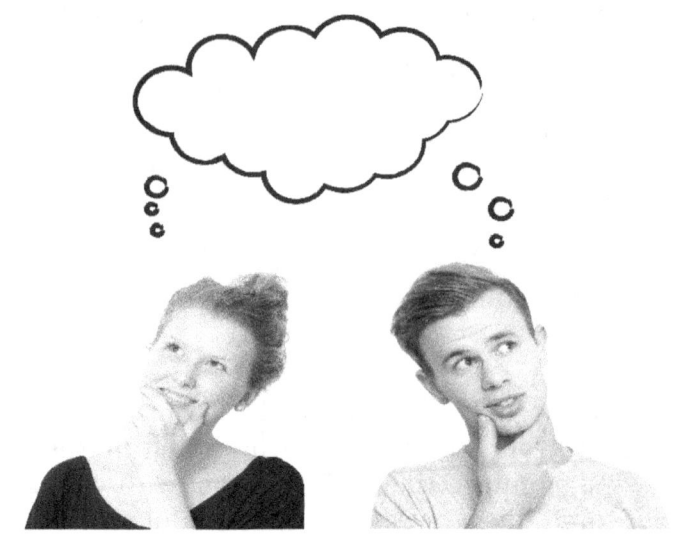

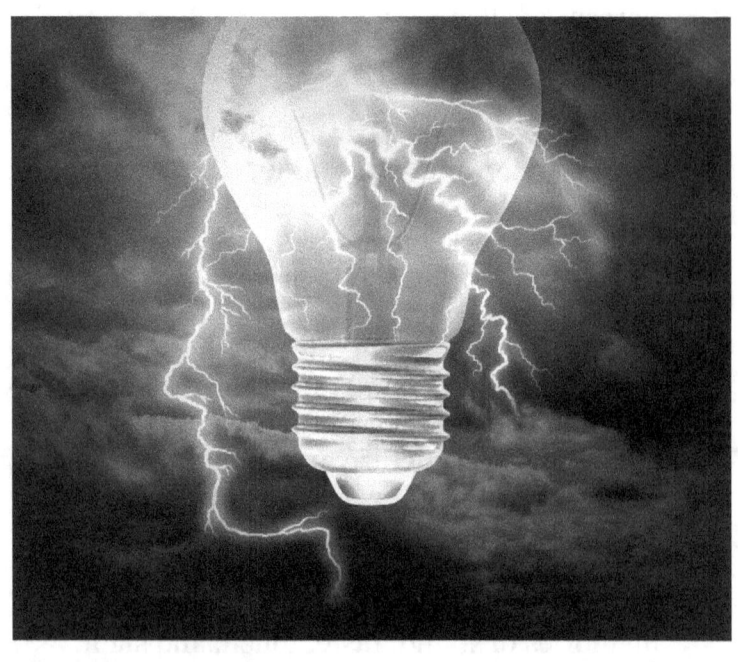

Cerebral Cortex

The cerebral cortex, which is as thick as a stack of two to three dimes, is an important tissue layer that coats the surface of the cerebellum and the cerebrum. In the cerebral cortex, the brain's actual information processing occurs. It is also considered the brain's 'gray matter.' It is colored gray since the area's nerves lack the insulation that makes the other brain parts seem white. The brain's folds add to the cortex's surface area and, thus, increase the amount of gray matter and the quantity of information that can be processed. The cerebral cortex includes three major areas, which serve as motor, sensory, and association hubs.

As is suggested by the name, the motor area plays a significant role in motion control-specifically, it governs our voluntary motions. It is the section of the cerebral cortex that enables us to properly perform the actions we desire to take.

The sensory hub is, naturally, responsible for processing much of the sense based input we receive on a daily basis. Vision, sound, and touch are all analyzed in this region. It enables us to process what we see and hear, and allows for all the sensations and experiences of touch.

The association area determines how we will perceive the world around us. It also allows us to plan our actions, engage in abstract thought, and learn, speak, and understand languages.

The Inner Brain

Within the brain are structures that function like gatekeepers between the cerebral hemispheres and the spinal cord. They determine your emotional state, modify responses and perceptions, and enable you to start movements without thinking. The structures are paired; each structure is duplicated in the opposite half of the brain.

About a pearl's size, the hypothalamus directs various significant functions. It is a vital emotional center as it controls the molecules that make you feel emotions of unhappiness, anger, or exhilaration. The hypothalamus is also your morning alarm clock and pumps up the adrenaline during a job interview or a test. It regulates when you feel hungry or tired, and even aids in the formation of bonds between humans, particularly familial ties. The thalamus, which is near the hypothalamus, is a

20

major processing center for information going from and to the cerebrum and the spinal cord. It processes visual, auditory, and tactile inputs and relays them to and from the appropriate zones. The thalamus also plays an important role in regulating our sleep cycles- to the extent that damage to the thalamus can cause a person to become unconscious or even comatose.

The hippocampus is a memory indexer, which is also a collection of nerve cells from the thalamus and the hypothalamus. It sends memories out to the cerebral hemisphere's relevant part for long-term storage and retrieving those memories when needed. Damage in this region can result in amnesia, and it is strongly linked to Alzheimer's and other memory-impairing conditions as well. The basal ganglia are nerve cell clusters that surround the thalamus. The basal ganglia initiate and integrate movements. The hippocampus also assists in movement and spatial awareness, enabling us to know where we are in our environment and how to navigate within it.

Connections

The nervous system and the brain are composed of various types of cells – just like any part of the human body. However, the basic functional unit of the CNS is the neuron. All movements, sensations, memories, feelings, and thoughts result from signals that pass through neurons.

Neurons have three basic parts: the cell body contains the nucleus, where nearly all of the molecules that the neuron requires to function and survive are produced. Dendrites branch out from the cell's body like tree branches and get messages from other nerve cells.

The signals pass from the dendrites to the cell body and they travel down an axon to a muscle cell, another neuron, or even cells in another organ. Support cells surround the neuron. There are some cells that surround the axon to form an insulating sheath, which can include myelin, which is a fatty molecule that insulates the axon and helps nerve signals to travel farther and faster.

The synapse is where signals travel from a neuron to a different cell. As the signal gets to the axon's end, it stimulates the discharge of tiny sacs, which release chemicals (neurotransmitters) into the synapse. Such neurotransmitters traverse the synapse and cling to receptors of the nearby cell. The receptors can also change the receiving cell's properties.

Working Neurotransmitters

Acetylcholine is an excitatory neurotransmitter because it causes cells to become more excitable. It causes glands to release hormones and it controls muscle contractions. A shortage of acetylcholine is linked to Alzheimer's disease.

Gamma-aminobutyric acid (GABA) is an inhibitory neurotransmitter since it causes cells to be less excitable. GABA is vital in the visual system and helps muscle activity control. Drugs to increase brain GABA level are used to treat tremors and epileptic seizures in Huntington's disease patients.

The neurotransmitter that brings on sleep and constricts blood vessels is serotonin, which also helps in temperature regulation. An inhibitory neurotransmitter, dopamine, is involved in movement control and mood. Dopamine activity loss in some of the brain's parts leads to Parkinson's disease's muscular rigidity.

Chapter 3: Geniuses and Average People

While the brain's anatomy is the same for every human being, there are a number of people who are intellectually advanced compared to the rest of the population. There are also a number of people who are deficient intellectually as well. What sets these people apart? Why are there geniuses and how are their brains different from the rest?

Throughout history, there have been people who have shown superior mental capabilities. People like Albert Einstein, Nikola Tesla, Leonardo da Vinci, Bobby Fischer, Ludwig van Beethoven, Madame Da Stael, and Marie Curie, among others. With the artistic and scientific contributions of such individuals throughout the centuries, the world has indeed become a better place.

It would be nice if we were able to become like them and come up with our own contribution to make the world even better, but, alas, that is not to be. Geniuses are a different breed, when it comes to variations in the brain's structure.

By what measure are geniuses considered what they are? While the above individuals and countless others have contributed greatly to society in terms of culture, science, and arts, there are still some questions. What makes them what they are? Are their brains different from the rest of us, the 'non-geniuses'?

Short and Long Connections

In a conventional human brain, there lies a relatively equal split from the short and long connections within the cerebral cortex. The short connections are linked to aptitude regarding to something that is of interest, while the long connections relate to the brain's capacity for things beyond such interests.

In the case of a genius's brain, the split between short and long connections normally leans more towards one connection or the other. Beethoven, for example, may have a good deal of cortical connections that are short; thus, hinting at his musical inclinations. Blaise Pascal, for example, may likely have more long cortical connections as he was accomplished highly in almost anything from prose to mathematics to philosophy.

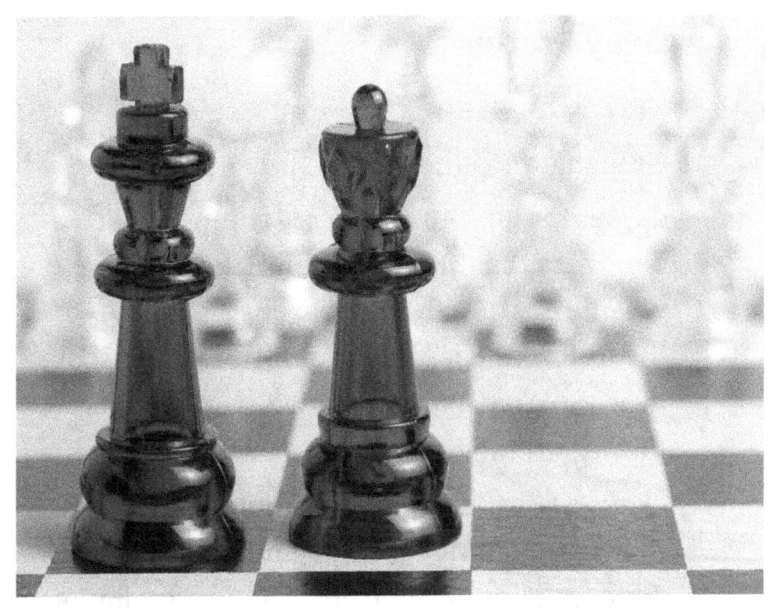

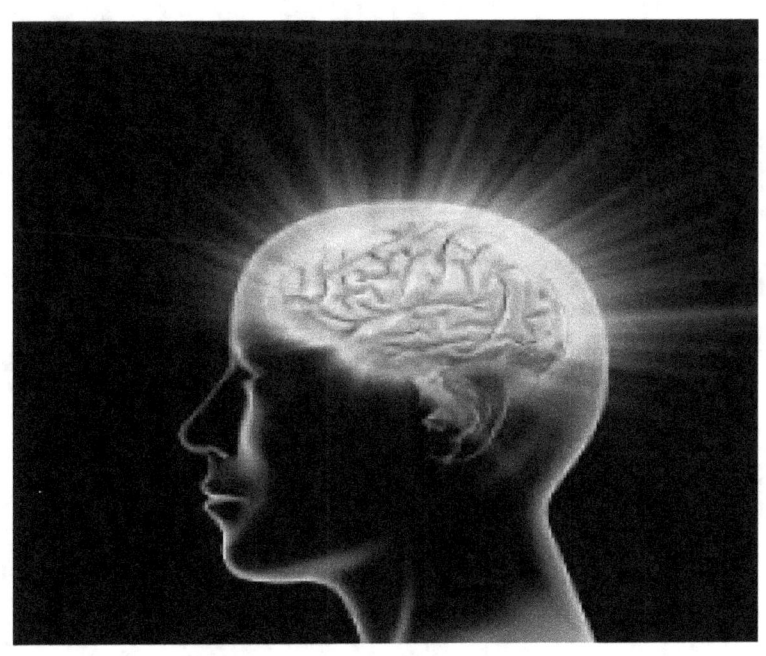

Gray Matter

Gray matter is the spinal cord and brain's darker tissue. Gray matter is composed of dendrites that branch out and literally wait to get information from the axons. In studies of the brains of people who gained high IQ scores, over 130 gray matter volumes were found. Moreover, the brain's white matter, where the axons are located, was also more substantial. The high quantity of white and gray matter nerve cells means that communication happens quickly and more effectively.

There have been recent publications of Albert Einstein's brain, which indicated that it not only had more and thicker gray matter, it also had more complex folds throughout Einstein's brain's gray matter. It also suggested that a lot of gray matter is an indication of a genius brain.

The Thalamus

The thalamus's dopamine receptors essentially determine what information goes through. The brain processes thoughts faster than we actually realize. The dopamine receptors and thalamus are basically the place where all thoughts converge. The valuable ones are able to go through, where the others are constricted and are more likely not able to reach conscious thought.

In a genius's brain, there are lesser dopamine receptors. Thus, the bottleneck is likely to be wider and allows more thoughts to pass through. Imagine the problem-solving and potential for creativity a person may have if more solutions and thoughts were allowed to come through.

The Genius's Approach

Since there may be tangible or physical characteristics in genius brains that are different from non-geniuses, there is also to be considered the genius's approach regarding thought in general. Imagine your method in approaching a problem. Maybe you begin with a lot of ideas. After that, you are likely to begin eliminating some of the ideas that don't seem to work, make sense, or suit the problem you're trying to solve.

A certain idea will not work because your funds may be limited. Another idea may also not work because you did it before and it did not succeed. Another idea of yours may not work out since nobody supported it. Gradually, you deliberate and eliminate your ideas and emerge with an idea or two that you think might succeed.

However, a genius's brain doesn't work that way. Ideas are not taken out based on practicality or efficacy. While everything is considered, thoughts are not disqualified immediately. Often, a genius attempts various methods to arrive at the desired outcome, instead of just deciding simply what ideas will or will not work.

A Long Way to Go

For a long time now, the term 'genius' has been used to classify someone who was especially adept or innovative. However, neuroscientists still face a long road ahead when it comes to finding out what sets genius brains apart from 'normal' people's brains. What seems to be clear is that there is no solitary factor that identifies it. Variances in the brain's thought processes and structure only comprise a portion of the puzzle. Trying to decide using that criterion alone will not suffice.

Chapter 4: Sharpening Your Brain

The body cannot function without the brain. The brain is what makes you move. It's what makes you feel. It's what makes you think. It's what helps you to sleep at night and wake up in the morning. The brain helps you to determine what foods you love to eat and what you want to throw away. It also determines if you are artistically inclined or whether you have great intellect.

Your thoughts are made in the brain, and the brain translates those thoughts into words or moves your body as you will it. As the pinnacle of intelligence, it is vital for you to keep the brain sharp so that you will stay rational and sane even until your old age.

As mentioned earlier, the brain is composed of several parts (the forebrain, the hindbrain, and the midbrain), with each part having different but very significant functions. For example, the midbrain controls reflex actions, eye movements, and some voluntary movements. The hindbrain controls bodily functions like respiration and heart rate.

The forebrain's substructures also hold highly significant functions and some of these substructures control your thoughts, emotions, and preferences. The frontal lobes allow you to deliberate the future, argue reasonably, and plan ahead. They are what make you rational. The parietal lobes allow you to enjoy the food you eat. You are also good at reading and mathematics because of your parietal lobes. The occipital lobes let you process images, while the temporal lobes allow you to swing to all kinds of music.

The substructures of the forebrain are not the only important components. Perhaps what supersedes such components is the gray matter or the cerebral cortex, where information processing occurs.

The brain's inner substructures are nevertheless important. The hypothalamus is your emotion center. The hippocampus is your memory indexer. The thalamus processes information passing through the spinal cord and the cerebrum. The basal ganglia integrate and start movements. Rounding up the brain's composite parts are the connectors and neurotransmitters. They complete the human being's nervous system.

Maintaining the health of the brain and the entire nervous system is important. Without a healthy brain and nervous system, how would you expect your body to function properly? There are many ways to keep the brain sharp. While this book presents 51 ways to sharpen your brain, there are many other things you can try.

When you use this book to help you to keep your brain alert, you do not do it with the intent to become a genius and suddenly compose a radical composition of music. You use the book not to become as intelligent as

Einstein and propose new theories. You do not use this book to become the next Leonardo da Vinci. You know that geniuses are a unique class of their own and their intelligence is somewhat difficult to emulate as explained earlier.

Instead, this book is a guide to help keep your brain sharp. The following chapter will show you how. It will show you what mind exercises you can do. It will also show you how you can keep your brain alert and active using various methods, which includes eating the right food, doing sufficient physical exercise, reading a lot, listening to music, and engaging in hobbies and activities.

While a lot of us may never become a genius like Einstein, you are at least assured that you can stay mentally alert, have a superior memory than the average crowd and that you can still do a lot of the things that you love to do as you grow older. You can at least assume that anyone can increase their brain power to some degree. Practicing the strategies described in this book can give you a hearty brainpower boost. They can also help you stay mentally healthy. Ultimately, the strategies mentioned here may help you to become considerably smarter.

Chapter 5: How to Boost Brain Power NATURALLY!

Now that we know all about the brain, its importance, how it functions, and what areas need to be touched so that it functions in an enhanced manner, let us go over some powerful techniques that will help us attain improved brain power, enhanced memory, intelligence, and concentration.

1. Brain exercises

Just like our body needs exercise to keep it fit and healthy, the brain also needs exercise. Brain exercises challenge the brain to think differently, think harder, or think fast. In short, you make the brain do something out-of-the-box. Regular exercise of the brain keeps it sharp, efficient and responsive. Exercises stimulate the brain to react quickly to situations and think faster than an average brain.

Here are some excellent brain exercises that can help you sharpen your brain power, improve memory, intelligence, concentration and focus.

Please do give them a try and see how your efficiency improves over time.

Exercise 1

Please get a notebook and a pen. Read the words written below in Italics (just once). After reading, turn to your notebook and start writing what you read. Write down everything that you remember. Your aim should be to write at least 14 of the 20 things that you read below. Here you go.

Bat, Hockey, Dollar, Mars, Mango,

Jeans, Truck, Sydney, Joker, James,

Yellow, Confidence, 5, Marriage, Wicket,

Man, Big Ben, Grass, Water, Magic.

Once you complete this task successfully, ask someone to write 20 new items and repeat the exercise.

This is a great exercise to train your brain to recall things.

Exercise 2

Please get a notebook and a pen. Think of a word ending with the letter 'e.' For example 'table.' Write it down on the notebook. Now, think of 9 other words ending with the letter 'e' and write them down.

When you are done, think and write down 9 words starting with the letter 'e.'

Let's now make it a bit more challenging. Think and write down a word ending with the letters 'a' and 't.' For example, 'fat'. Now write down 9 words ending with the letters 'a' and 't'.

Please come up with your own permutations and combinations and continue the exercise for a few minutes.

Doing this at least once a day will train your brain to think in a disciplined way.

Exercise 3

Sit down in a quiet place with a pen and paper. Go back to one of your oldest memories – a picnic, a wedding, or even some celebration at home. Start writing about the event describing what happened.

Be as specific as possible with complete details right down to the color of the clothes worn that day. You may not remember it distinctly but think hard and if the event is really close to your heart, you will be amazed how pictures of the event will flash in front of your eyes.

Try and write for as long as possible and, once done, keep it aside. Writing is a great exercise for the brain. When you write about an old memory, you are churning the brain, not just making it go back and forth, but also persuading it to express the memory in words.

A day later, read what you had written and enjoy the smile on your face!

You should do this exercise at least once every two weeks. This will not just exercise your brain but it is also a wonderful stress-reliever.

Exercise 4

Close the door of your room and put on some loud music – just loud enough for yourself and not for anyone outside your room. Please get a book, a magazine, or a newspaper. Select a paragraph with at least 5 lines in it. Now, read and try to memorize it. The music should be on continuously.

This is an excellent way of training the brain to concentrate. Most people are not able to study or do their work when there is a lot of chaos around. This is because the brain is not able to shut out what is not required.

Doing this exercise daily will help you make the brain focus on what is required and ignore what is not.

Exercise 5

Juggling with balls in hand for 10 minutes every-day is a good exercise for the brain. Start with 2 balls and go on to 3. Juggling with 4 balls can be really tough so you can stick to 3.

Keep 2 balls in your right hand and 1 in your left hand. Throw one ball from the right hand into the air and catch it with the left hand. Before your catch while the ball is in the air, pass on the ball which is in your left hand to the right hand so the right hand now has 2.

Repeat the cycle. Look to increase the speed with every passing minute. Do not worry if the balls keep falling. It will take some practice.

This exercise will improve your concentration and focus tremendously.

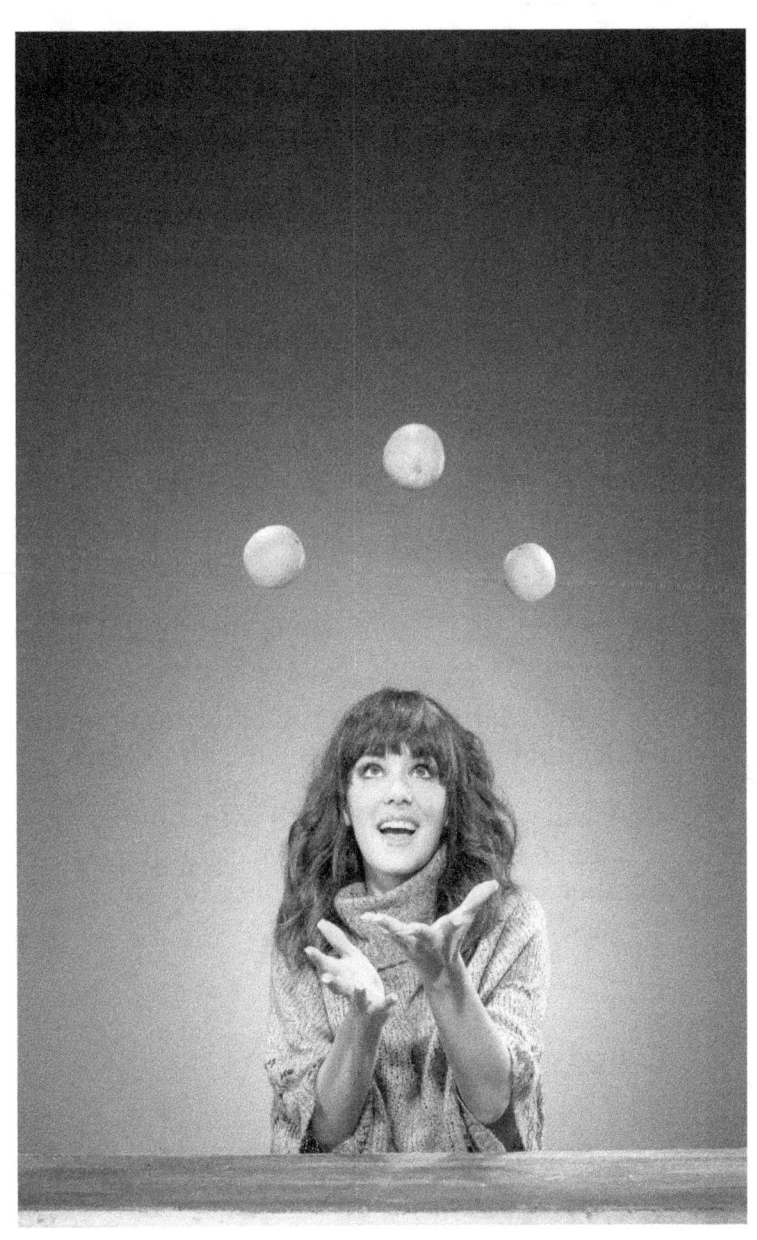

Exercise 6

Put on your headsets and listen to a completely new song. Halfway through the song, switch it off and try singing that song recalling the lyrics. Recall and sing as much as you can.

Music has an excellent soothing effect on the brain. When you listen to something new, you are stimulating the brain. When you ask the brain to recall it immediately after, you are giving it a fabulous dose of work-out.

Exercise 7

Solve this Mathematics problem without using a calculator and with just a pen and paper.

How will you get a total of 18 with numbers 3, 6, 4 and 9 using +, -, ×, ÷. You can use the numbers and the signs only once for this exercise.

Exercise 8

Counting the number of times the letter 'f' appears in a sentence is beneficial.

Let's take this example - the sentence is,

"Finished files are the result of years of scientific study combined with the experience of years."

Did you count three 'f,' or six? There are six of them in the sentence. Why is this so? The brain seemingly cannot process correctly the word 'OF.' The letter 'f' seems to make the 'f' sound, similar to 'forest.' In the word 'OF,' however, the 'f' makes a 'v' sound. Thus, the brain seems to overlook 'of' as it searches for the sound of 'f.'

Exercise 9

Here is an activity to exercise your parietal lobes (visual interpretation) and frontal lobes (attention and working memory). Quickly count as fast as you can as to how many times the figure '6' appears in the numerical group below.

Afterwards, count up how many times the figures '3' and '7' appear below. Try to sum up the total of both numbers once you finish counting. Don't do this by first counting the 3s and then the 7s. Count them as your eyes scan over them.

123446788997467465786587 6576576

3576573625432657346578436578342

2732188582735827456724687343828

767287868276872368237 6783768267

2647648823178346432764876774653

7436574386581483627868653873465

Getting the accurate answer is not important here, but the attempt is. For decades, such exercise has been used by militaries for attention improvement. While there are now better ways of improving attention like using computer-based advanced tools, this exercise is fun.

Exercise 10

Solving riddles is also an excellent way to keep your brain sharp. Try to guess this riddle.

"A blind beggar had a brother who died. What relation was the blind beggar to the brother who died?"

Did you answer 'brother?' No, it's not the correct answer. The answer is 'sister.' The blind beggar is a female, thus, she is the 'sister' of the dead man. Why? The riddle baffles anyone who has not heard it before, even though it is stated simply. Since the listener has a tendency to assume implicitly about gender, the listener may assume that the blind beggar is male.

How is the brain exercised? The riddle delves on analytical functions like hypothesis testing, abstract reasoning, and implicit assumptions in the frontal lobes. It also tests emotional memory as well as creativity in finding unique solutions to problems.

Exercise 11

Exercise your brain for the weekend to train working memory and attention.

- Backwards, say the days of the week. Also say them in alphabetical order.

- In alphabetical order, say the year's months. If you think it is easy, try saying them in reverse alphabetical order (now that's really tough!).

- For each letter in your full name, mention two objects. Work up to a maximum of five objects while trying to come up with different items every time.

- What is the sum of your birth date, mm/dd/yyyy? You can also do the same with your other relatives or friends.

- In your location and within 2 minutes, look around. Try to look for five red objects that you can put in your pocket. Also look for five blue objects that are too large to fit in your pocket.

Exercise 12

Enrolling in a cooking class is an excellent brain exercise. Plus, you also get to learn new cuisines.

Cooking requires a number of senses. All senses involve various parts of the brain and hence it is a great exercise.

Exercise 13

Drawing a map from memory is another excellent way to exercise your brain.

When you come home from a new place, try to draft a map or plan of the place you visited. Do this exercise each time you go to a new location.

Exercise 14

Indulge in Brain aerobics. They can be as simple as doing crossword puzzles, intellectually-charged board games, thinking of famous people and celebrities whose first names start with a letter 'a.' etc.

Even surfing the Internet activates brain regions related to complex reasoning and decision-making. Thus, unlike watching TV, browsing the Internet is a stimulating task that could really help you to boost brainpower.

2. Meditation

One of the most powerful and natural ways of improving brain power is through daily meditation. Today, modern science tells us through various studies that meditation has the power to improve those areas of the brain, which are connected to raw intelligence, memory, and awareness. Meditation improves the frequency of the brain waves leading to higher levels of relaxation, concentration, and focus when doing any task.

Research shows how people who have been meditating for years have a far more developed brain and increased grey matter. Normally as the years pass, the brain tends to show down, but if one is meditating daily, the brain continues to maintain the same level of intensity. You can thus be on par not just with your children but also your grand-children when it comes to grasping new technologies for instance.

There are several methods of meditating that can be done at any time during the day. However the best time to meditate is in the morning as soon as you get up. Before you get soaked into the routines of the day, soak yourself first in meditation.

Here is a simple way to meditate:

Choose a quiet place where there are no distractions. Sit cross legged with your palms on the knees facing upwards. You can also sit on a chair if that is more comfortable. The most important thing to know is to keep your back (the vertebral column) straight throughout.

Close your eyes and start breathing normally keeping your head straight.

Now, focus your attention on your breath and feel it going in and out. Breathing should only be through your nose and not the mouth. You will notice that time and again your focus shifts from your breath towards your thoughts. Do not worry. This is normal especially if you are new to meditation. Just do this - as soon as you become aware that your focus has shifted from your breath to your thoughts, pull yourself back to your breath.

Keep doing this for at least 5 minutes and gradually increase your time over a period of days. Your goal should be to do a minimum of 15 minutes of this exercise every day in the morning. You will notice that with regular practice, your focus will settle on your breath and your mind will stop wandering to different things; and that is Meditation.

You should try and make meditation a part of your daily routine. Slowly but surely the ability to focus during meditation will come naturally to you. In fact once you have meditated for a couple of weeks, you will be amazed how you will start enjoying it. You will not want to start your day without it. So just go for it.

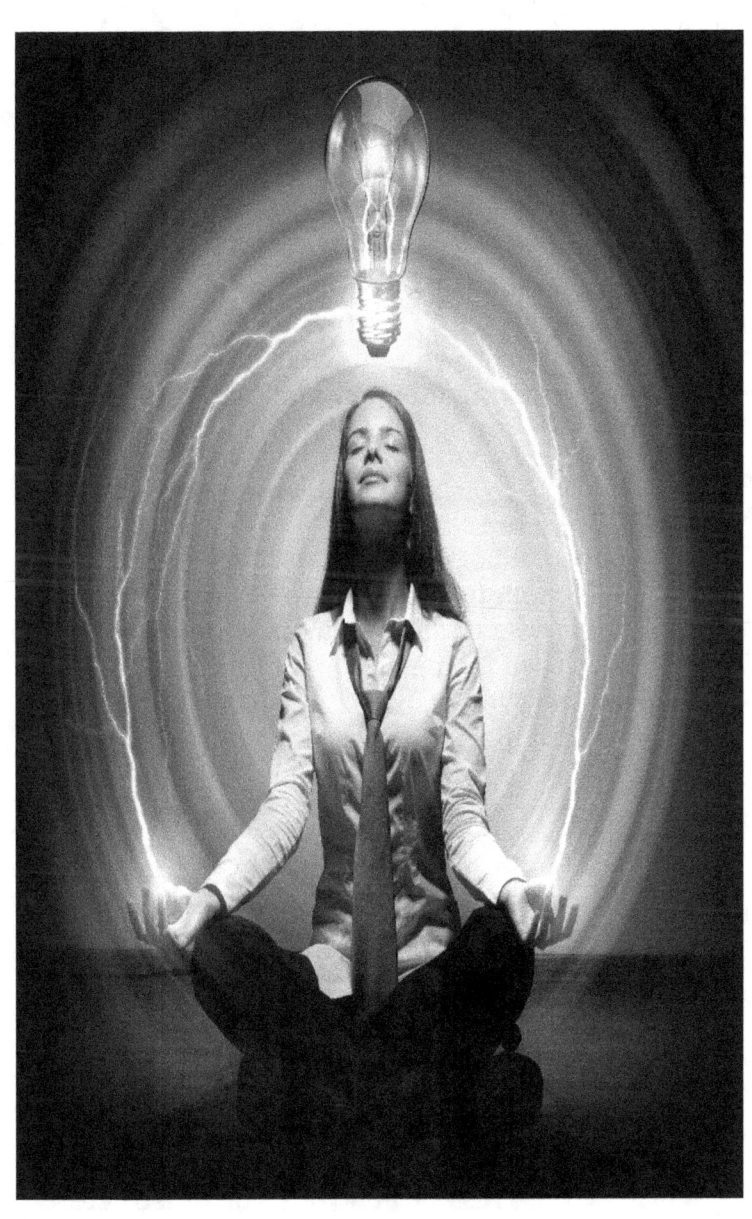

3. Sirsasana (Headstand)

Sirsasana or Headstand is a yoga position wherein the body is inverted and held straight up with the head resting on the floor lightly supported by forearms. Since the body is turned upside down, there is an increased flow of blood into the brain. This provides greater levels of oxygen to the brain and also helps the brain to absorb vital nutrients in a huge way thus improving memory and other functions of the brain.

If you are a beginner, Sirsasana should be practiced under the guidance of a qualified Yoga instructor as you do not want to injure yourself practicing alone. Along with the instructor, you can also use a wall for balance. Below are the steps to perform Sirsasana:

- Sit in a kneeling position.

- Place your elbows on the floor. Then rest your head lightly on the floor.

- Push forward and move your buttocks up. This is when your Yoga Instructor needs to help you maintain your balance.

- Slowly move your legs up ensuring the body weight is on your forearms and not on the head.

- Straighten your legs and ensure the entire body is straight. This is the final position. Stay like this for a minute and then come out of the pose by reversing the steps mentioned above. It will take a few days for you to master the steps. Once you come out of Sirsasana, lie down on the floor with both your body and head facing up towards the ceiling. Do this for 2 minutes to ensure even distribution of the blood in the body.

You can begin doing Sirsasana initially for a couple of minutes and then gradually increase the time. You can go up to 15 to 20 minutes per session. You should be on an empty stomach and hence the best time to practice this exercise is mornings; before breakfast and after you have emptied your bowels.

If you are doing meditation, it is recommended that you do Sirsasana before meditation for maximum benefits. Regular and proper practice of both meditation and Sirsasana can do wonders for the brain and you will see how your ability to concentrate and focus on your work improves tremendously over a period of time.

You should avoid Sirsasana if you are suffering from head, neck or any other body injury. Also people with high blood pressure, heart condition and brain or eye injury should not perform Sirsasana. If you have any other medical condition, please consult your doctor before attempting Sirsasana.

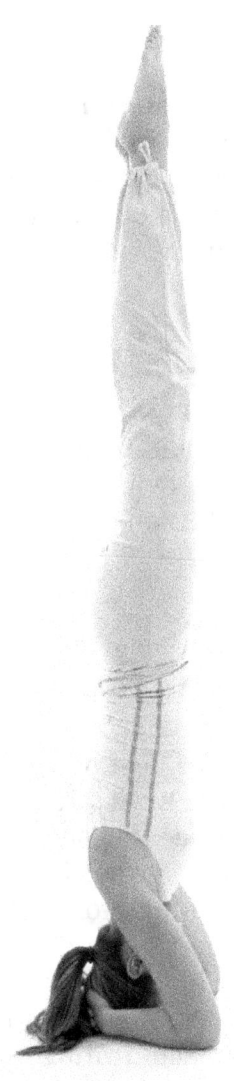

Improving Memory Through Nutrition

You can improve your brainpower by eating the right kinds of food. Here are some of your favored drinks, food, nutritional supplements, flavorings, and condiments that nourish your brain so that it can operate clearly and quickly, as it should.

The good thing is that these foods can just be found in your pantry. You don't have to go the fancy health food store and buy products with ingredients from the Amazon.

4. Honey

Honey is one of the oldest natural foods, which was also used as a natural sweetener for centuries before processed sugar was invented. The process by which honey is made by honey-bees makes it one of the most nutritional foods with medicinal properties in it as well. A teaspoon of honey in your daily food can do wonders for your brain boosting memory, intelligence, and concentration power.

Honey being full of antioxidants, daily consumption helps to keep the cells in the brain intact and prevents damage of any kind. Various studies have been conducted over the years to understand the effect of honey. Results have shown that honey not just aids in improving memory but also helps in developing the nervous system thus reducing stress and anxiety.

There are various ways in which honey can be made part of your daily diet. You can either have a teaspoon of it directly or mix it with milk and have it along with your break-fast in the morning. Honey if consumed with milk just before going to bed aids in restful sleep and helps the brain relax so that it is stress-free the next day morning.

Studies have shown that daily consumption of honey helps to improve learning abilities and also enhances intellectual capacity in later life.

Honey should not be given to newborns until they are over 12 months as it can lead to infant botulism. Refer to the instructions on the label or check with your doctor before administering honey to kids.

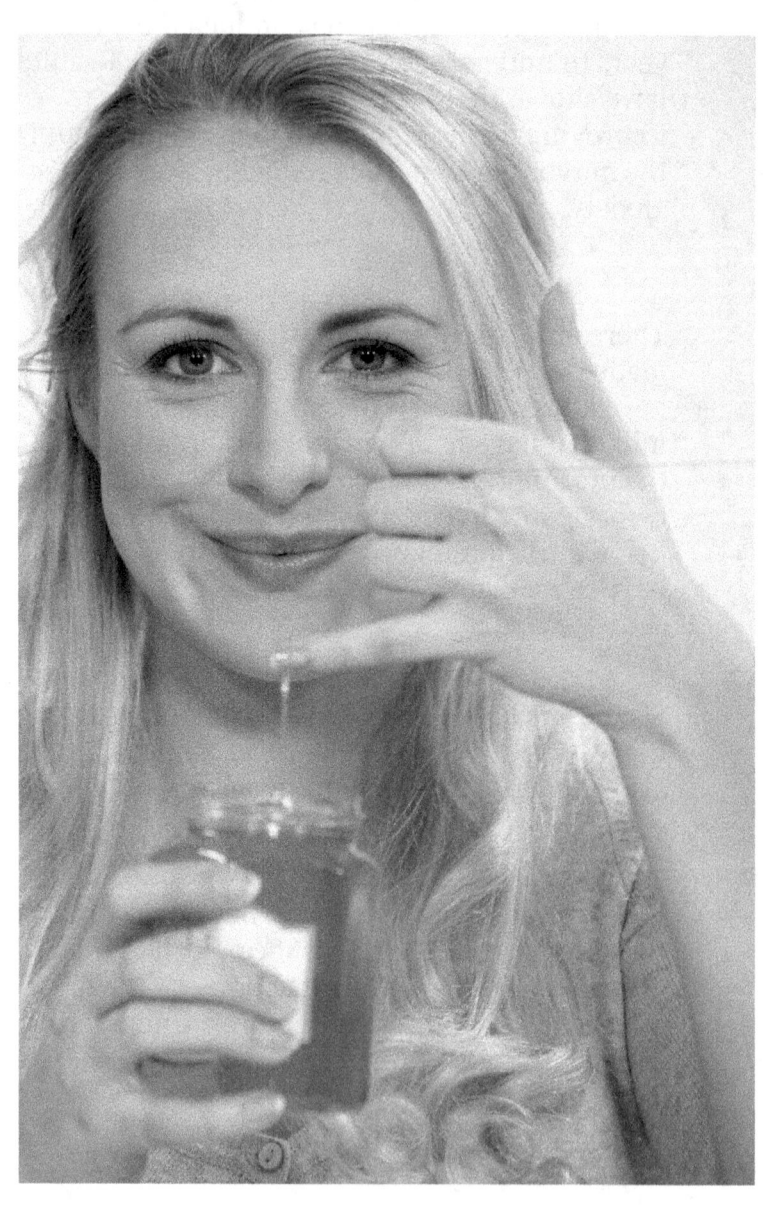

5. Rosemary

For a long time now, this condiment has been tied with memory improvement. Rosemary has considerable anti-inflammatory and antioxidant properties to stave off free radical damage in the brain.

Rosemary enhances both concentration and memory. After all, after what William Shakespeare wrote about rosemary, "There's rosemary, that's for remembrance," you would surely want to enhance the flavor of your food with this memory-enhancing ingredient.

6. Berries

While all kinds of berries are beneficial for the brain, blueberries are considered to be the best "brain food." Berries, especially blueberries, have compounds called anthocyanins, which have been linked to memory improvement.

Berries are also linked to the improvement of other cognitive skills like reasoning, learning, verbal comprehension, numerical ability, and decision making.

7. Nuts

All the varieties of nuts are rich in B-complex vitamins, omega-3 fatty acids, vitamin E, zinc, iron, and magnesium.

All of nuts' nutrients are essential for the brain. However, walnuts stand above the rest of the nuts as they are good at preventing brain aging and they also improve memory.

A fun thing to note is that a walnut closely resembles a brain.

8. Curry

Curries are a blend of spices like black pepper and turmeric that synergistically work to promote memory improvement and to make you smart too.

The turmeric's curcumin component is what makes curry good for your brain. Turmeric's component can easily cross the barrier that divides the blood and the brain.

9. Avocados

Avocados are considered the "world's most perfect food." It can help stave off Alzheimer's disease and it boosts production of dopamine, a neurotransmitter that helps you to stay focused.

The creamy avocado is also rife with vitamins and fiber. However, what makes it valuable as brain food is that the avocado is a source of healthy fats.

10. Chocolate

Chocolate has flavonoids, when combined with theobromine and caffeine; they create a feeling that is similar to being in love. The flavonoids in chocolate also contribute to improved attention, focus, and memory that chocolate aficionados get to experience.

Chocolate can also be enjoyed as a drink. It has been noted that elders (seniors) improve their memories for a few hours after drinking hot chocolate. Dark chocolate is best for the brain as the presence of milk binds with some of chocolate's beneficial compounds.

You must however note that over-indulgence of anything is not good and hence you must consume chocolate in moderation.

11. Water

Get hydrated and stay hydrated. While water composes 75% of the human brain, many of us are dehydrated chronically. Even mild dehydration leads to brain tissue shrinkage and momentary loss of cognitive function.

There are also studies on today's water supply that contains fluoride; studies suggest that the fluoride in our drinking water lowers IQ. The solution is that if your water supply has fluoride, make sure to install a filter, which takes away fluoride.

12. Coconut Oil

Once considered as unhealthy, new studies suggest that coconut oil is indeed healthy and is beneficial for the brain. Coconut oil has MCTs (medium chain triglycerides) that nourish the brain through bypassing the metabolism of glucose.

Coconut oil is normally used in cooking. Plus, it may even help warding off Alzheimer's disease. MCTs are now even found in Alzheimer's patients' prescription-only food.

13. Wild-Caught Salmon

Wild-caught salmon, free-range eggs and poultry and pasture-raised pork are excellent sources for omega-3 fatty acids, which are some of the brain's most important nutrients.

Include Salmon in your diet but ensure it is wild caught and not farmed.

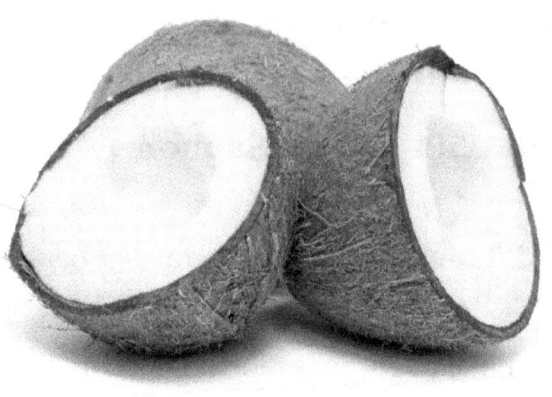

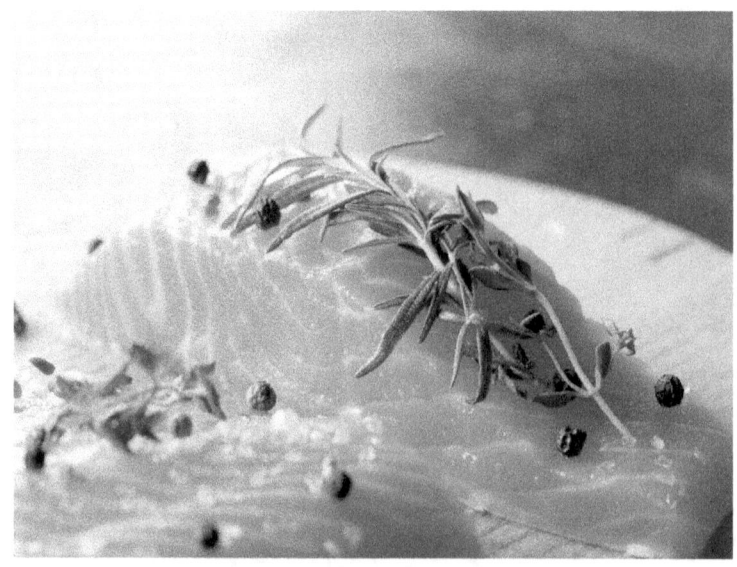

14. Yerba Mate

Derived from a member of the holly family, yerba mate is a traditional tea from South America.

Drinkers of yerba mate tea report increased focus, clarity, and increased mental energy, but without the jitters that usually accompany doses of caffeine. Author Tim Ferriss considers yerba mate to be his favored brain-boosting drink.

15. Green Tea

Green tea is an excellent source of l-theanine, which is an amino acid that may improve mood, learning, and memory recall. Combined with caffeine (also found in green tea), l-theanine has a synergistic effect, which boosts the function of the brain.

L-theanine also hinders the buildup of brain plaque, which makes green tea a preventative drink against Alzheimer's disease.

16. Coffee

Aside from its brain-boosting properties, coffee is the world's most popular substance. As a brain booster, coffee improves mood, overall brain function, and memory. For the long haul, coffee can also help keep your memory sharp. What makes it even better is that coffee can also greatly reduce the risk of Alzheimer's disease.

You must however enjoy coffee in moderation as too much of it can make you get addicted to it.

17. Apples and Bananas

Both apples and bananas are hugely rich in nutrients. As it is said, 'an apple a day keeps the doctor away', the same goes for banana too. Apart from keeping the doctors away, both these fruits are very good food for the brain and supply them with vital nutrients.

18. Vitamins C and E

The combination of Vitamin C and Vitamin E is promising for the improvement of memory.

The combination synergistically works to improve memory. The combination also helps to lower the risk of developing dementia and Alzheimer's disease by 60%.

Vitamin C can be found in all citrus fruits and also in tomatoes, pineapples and leafy vegetables. You can get Vitamin E in nuts, blackberries, avocados, olive oil and spinach.

19. Vitamin B12

In the United States, the most common vitamin deficiency is Vitamin B12 deficiency. This deficiency can lead to a number of disorders, dementia being one of them.

Vitamin B12 can be easily found in fish, eggs, poultry and meat.

20. Vitamin D

Vitamin D is created when your body is exposed to the sun. This Vitamin can increase your problem-solving ability, improve memory, banish depression, and lift your mood.

Exposing yourself to the sun whenever you can is the easiest and best way to get Vitamin D. Early morning sun is the best source. However, if sunlight is a rarity (especially in northern climates), you should eat foods which contain Vitamin D such as salmon, tuna, mackerel, mushrooms and fortified milk.

21. DHA (docosahexaenoic acid)

As a type of omega-3 fatty acid, DHA is essential as your brain's building block. DHA has been proven to boost mood and improve memory. Studies show that people with dementia, ADHD, or Alzheimer's have been found to improve with DHA supplementation.

DHA can be found in animal products such as meat and eggs. Fish such as salmon and mackerel are also a good source.

22. Avoid Low-Fat Diets

Low-fat diets do not do you any favors when it comes to weight loss and they can spell disaster for our brains. They may even contribute to the rise of Alzheimer's cases.

The brain has 60 percent fat, and it contains around 25% of the body's cholesterol content. The lack of good cholesterol increases the likelihood of dementia, depression, and suicide. Thus, high cholesterol (the good kind) reduces dementia risk.

23. Avoid Sugar or at Least Reduce Your Intake

It is established that sugar is harmful to the brain. However, many people still consume pounds and pounds of it.

What does refined sugar do to the brain? It leads to depression, learning disorders, and poor memory formation. Constant levels of high body sugar can lead to decreased activity of the hippocampus, which is linked to memory. Excess body sugar affects short-term memory, mood stability, and attention span.

24. Avoid MSG (monosodium glutamate)

MSG, like artificial sugar, breaks down into glutamate (a known excitotoxin) and formaldehyde.

MSG can lead to digestive upset, asthma, mood swings, migraines, and brain fog.

Unfortunately, MSG is found in most processed foods and is certainly hard to avoid. Normally, if the food is salty, chances are it has a lot of MSG. Some of the offending food products include noodles, refined soy products, snack foods, and canned soups.

25. Avoid Microwave Popcorn (butter-flavored)

Don't add the butter flavoring to your microwave popcorn. Better yet, avoid microwave popcorn altogether.

The butter flavoring has diacetyl (an additive) that causes beta-amyloid clamping in your brain. This can raise your risk of developing Alzheimer's.

26. Avoid Drinking Diet Soda

Diet products, especially diet soda, have artificial sweeteners. Aspartame, an artificial sweetener, breaks down into excitotoxins and formaldehyde. The excitotoxins stimulate or literally 'excite' brain cells to death.

Although sucralose (another artificial sweetener used more frequently these days) is a lesser evil than aspartame, prolonged intake of it can lead to migraines, headaches, brain fog, dizziness, tinnitus, depression, and anxiety.

Physical Exercise to Benefit Your Brain

Aside from benefiting our bodies, physical exercise also keeps our brains healthy and fit. Physical exercise is considered even more beneficial than thinking and is the best thing that can help keep your brain health. The best kinds of physical exercise that benefit your brain directly are enjoyable and can help to improve your memory.

27. Qi Gong and Tai Chi

Qi gong and tai chi entail a sequence of movements performed in a focused and slow manner, which are accompanied by deep breaths. This ancient oriental physical exercise can be done easily and can give your body and brain an excellent workout. They can help improve thinking ability and memory.

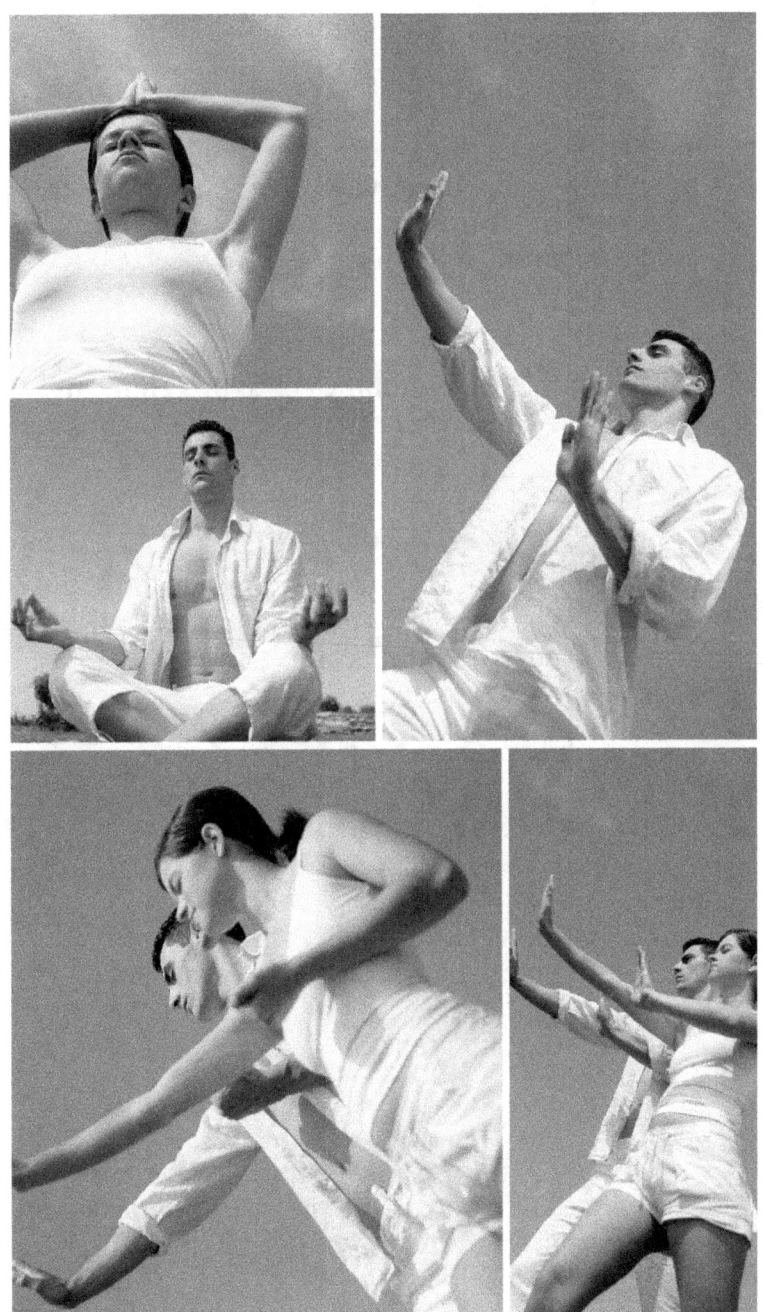

28. Yoga

Mentioned earlier is sirasana, which is a specific yoga pose, to help keep the brain sharp. However, sirasana is only one facet of yoga among many other poses.

Generally, yoga combines both breathing and poses to balance and strengthen your mind and body.

The benefits of yoga to your brain health include better sleep, stress reduction, and better mood, mental balance, and concentration.

29. Exercise Outdoors

Compared with indoor exercise, outdoor exercise increases enthusiasm, vitality, self-esteem, and pleasure, while lowering fatigue, depression, and tension.

After an hour of being surrounded by nature, your attention span and memory performance can improve by 20%.

One of the brain's best overall exercises is gardening. This is why people who love gardening tend to have lower risk of dementia than non-gardeners.

30. Walking for Brain Health

Walking is one of the best exercises for getting a clear mind. While 10,000 steps daily are desirable, most people on average walk for about 3,000 steps daily.

To make sure you get your 10,000 steps, it is best for you to have an activity tracking device. For instance, you can use pedometers to determine how many steps you have taken and thus make adjustments if necessary.

31. Stand Up Often

The human body is designed to move a lot. However, many people spend around 12 hours a day sitting. Plus, the extended sitting makes us sluggish and sick, physically and mentally.

The cure for such sluggishness is not walking or more exercise. The answer is standing up.

According to Dr. Joan Vernikos, an ex-NASA physician, the solution is to frequently stand up throughout the day. This should be done at least 30 times.

Other Brain Workouts

As the brain benefits from physical exercise, mental exercises also help a lot. It doesn't mean you have to constantly answer riddles or take visual exams or abstract reasoning tests. Any activity that is challenging, fun, and new can be considered as a 'brain' workout.

Benefits include improved mood and memory, faster thinking, better hearing and vision, better reaction time, and feelings of increased productivity, motivation, and focus.

The secret is to keep things fun and engaging so you will do it more often.

32. Indulge in a Hobby

Crafts and hobbies like woodworking or knitting can be considered brain exercises as well since they help us focus, much like meditation.

Hobbies are natural anti-depressants and could protect you from premature brain aging.

Research indicates that 'purposeful activities' like crafts, arts, and doing home repairs especially stimulate the nervous system and improve mental well-being as well.

33. Listen to Music

One of the few activities that require the simultaneous use of the brain's two sides is listening to music.

Listening to music, especially instrumental music, can lead to improved attention and focus, memory, physical coordination, and language skills.

Playing an instrument is even better for development compared to just listening to music passively. Whether it is dancing, singing, playing, or listening to music, it is beneficial to your brain one way or another.

34. Having Purpose in Life

A clearly-defined life purpose can decrease your risk of developing Alzheimer's in the future. Plus, people who pursue their passion live longer, have better mental health, and are happier.

Having a purpose helps in planning your life. Even though things may not always turn out the way you had planned but if you have your life vision and purpose in place, your ability to swing back and re-plan is better than those who just live life as it happens to them.

The brain is far more active when there is a clear purpose attached to one's existence.

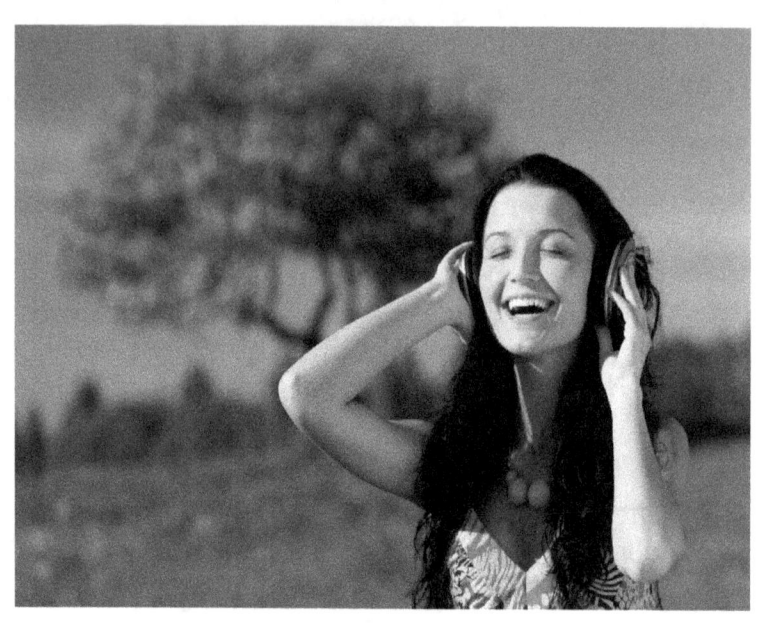

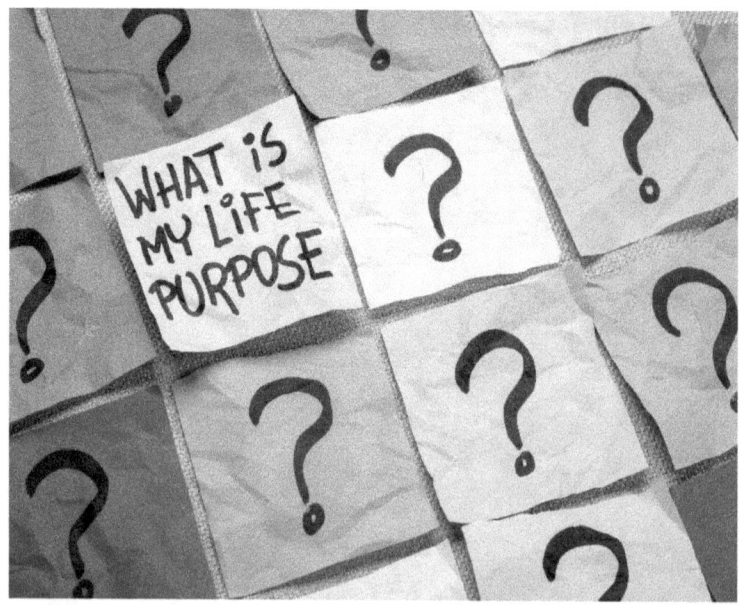

35. Learn Something New

One of the easiest ways to boost brainpower is to keep on learning new things. The neurons' structure and size and the connections that link them really change as you learn.

Some ways of challenging your mind include participating in community and social activities or even playing an instrument. Or perhaps just learn a new skill. No matter what new stuff you want to do, the important thing to know is that, when the learning process stops, some of your brain's parts begin to atrophy. Plus, neural connections that are not used start to wither away.

Good thing for us living in this century is that there is a wide avenue for learning. The Internet has made a whole lot of knowledge available for you. Websites like Udemy and Khan Academy have more than enough online learning tools to last you a long time.

36. Be Creative

Embrace your hidden artistic talent. Creating any kind of art makes you more observant, stimulates your imagination, and promotes memory improvement.

Art therapy can improve Alzheimer's patients' memories by up to 70%. Art therapy can also boost cognitive abilities in people, even those who have serious conditions.

37. Reduce the Usage of GPS

Relying heavily on GPS technology use is causing us to be mentally lazy. Doing so also destroys our natural navigation skills, which have taken humans millennia to perfect.

Use a map. Learn how to read it. It is said that in order to stimulate his mind, Bill Gates uses different driving routes to and from his house every day. No wonder he is doing so well even now when he's retired.

38. Learn to Speak Another Language

A bilingual person is already better off than the rest of the population. This is because speaking more languages is one of the more practical and effective ways to keep your mind sharp and retain memory.

Learning a new language can protect you from age-related mental decline, improve your cognitive skills, and eventually make you smarter. And yes, it requires a lot of effort to learn a new language so it is a great way to exercise the brain cells.

39. Go on a Vacation

Travelling to new places is one of the rare life experiences that can stimulate your brain and stretch your mind. However, vacation days can go unused if a person is very busy with work. Do yourself, and your brain, a favor. Go on a vacation and leave work behind; come home rejuvenated and mentally stimulated – and see how your productivity improves.

You should try and visit different places and see the different cultures across the world. Experiencing the diversity is a wonderful way to broaden your thinking.

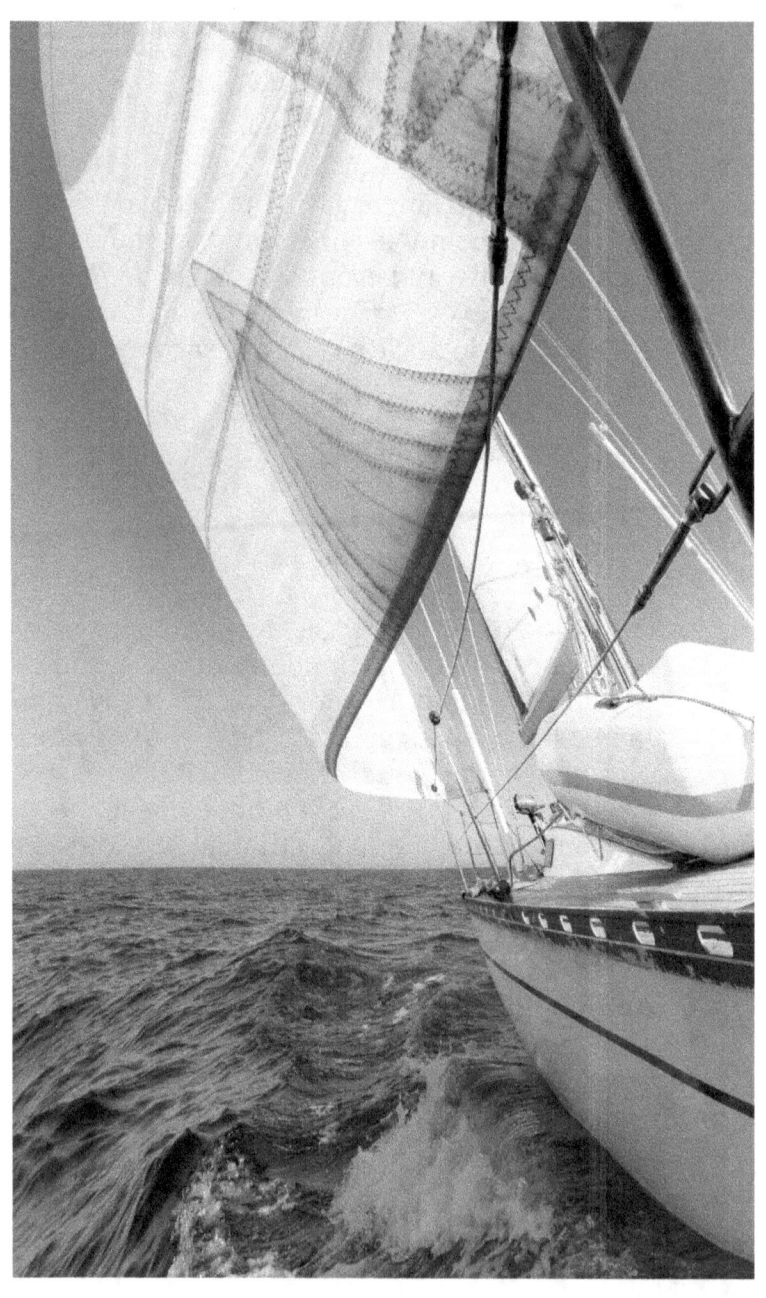

40. Read a Good Book

Reading a book, or a magazine, is one of the best ways to activate your brain. Reading a book reduces stress, improves analytical thinking and memory, and increases intelligence.

The more you write and read, the better off your brain will be as you grow older and wiser.

41. Try 'Neurobics'

What is neurobics? The term was coined by Dr. Lawrence Katz in his book 'Keep Your Brain Alive: 83 Neurobic Exercises to Help Prevent Memory Loss and Increase Mental Fitness.'

Some examples of Neurobic exercises are wearing your watch in reverse, utilizing your non-dominant hand, eating with chopsticks, or folding laundry with closed eyes.

Unique Ways to Improve Memory

Besides physical exercise, mental exercise, and eating right, there are many other ways to improve brain health.

Some of the unique ways to improve memory include seemingly unrelated items like your mobile phone or body parts like your stomach or even your weight.

Below are some different ways to make your brain do some work.

42. Reduce Multitasking

A multitasking attempt affects the way you remember, concentrate, and learn. Multitasking can even prematurely age your brain cells by shortening the 'telomeres,' which are protective end caps on your chromosomes.

Anyway, it is impossible to do many tasks at once. The brain toggles quickly between tasks and sacrifices the efficiency of doing a particular task for another.

If you are trying to impress your boss with your multitasking powers, think again.

43. Eliminate Clutter

With the use of MRI (magnetic resonance imaging), researchers have found out that clutter does affect how your brain processes information and how it concentrates.

An organized environment can make you more productive and focused, and you get to remember information when you need it. Plus, an organized environment improves your mood.

44. Challenge Negative Thinking

In a day, an average person has about 50,000 thoughts. However, a lot of them are negative. Your thoughts create your brain. They are not merely fleeting moments created inside your brain. Positive thoughts shape your brain in a positive way. You should therefore think more positively than negatively.

Thoughts can change your brain by stimulating neurotransmitter production. The neurotransmitters can change the function and structure of your brain. Whether that change is positive or negative depends on you – so choose to think positively and see the bright side of things, accentuate the positive!

45. Balance Intestinal Flora

Your gut health affects your brain, surprisingly. Bad bacteria proliferation increases brain inflammation, disrupts neurotransmitter balance, and damages your memory seat – the hippocampus.

Serotonin, which is the 'happy' neurotransmitter, is mostly created in your gut. Good bacteria should flourish in your gut and you can do this by eating fermented food like raw sauerkraut, kefir, and yogurt. A good probiotic supplement is good if you have digestive issues.

46. Enjoy Time with Friends

An active social life leads to a slow mental decline. Even a 10-minute conversation with a friend everyday can do wonders.

A good laugh with your friend is even better since laughter can increase memory ability by reducing cortisol – the stress hormone.

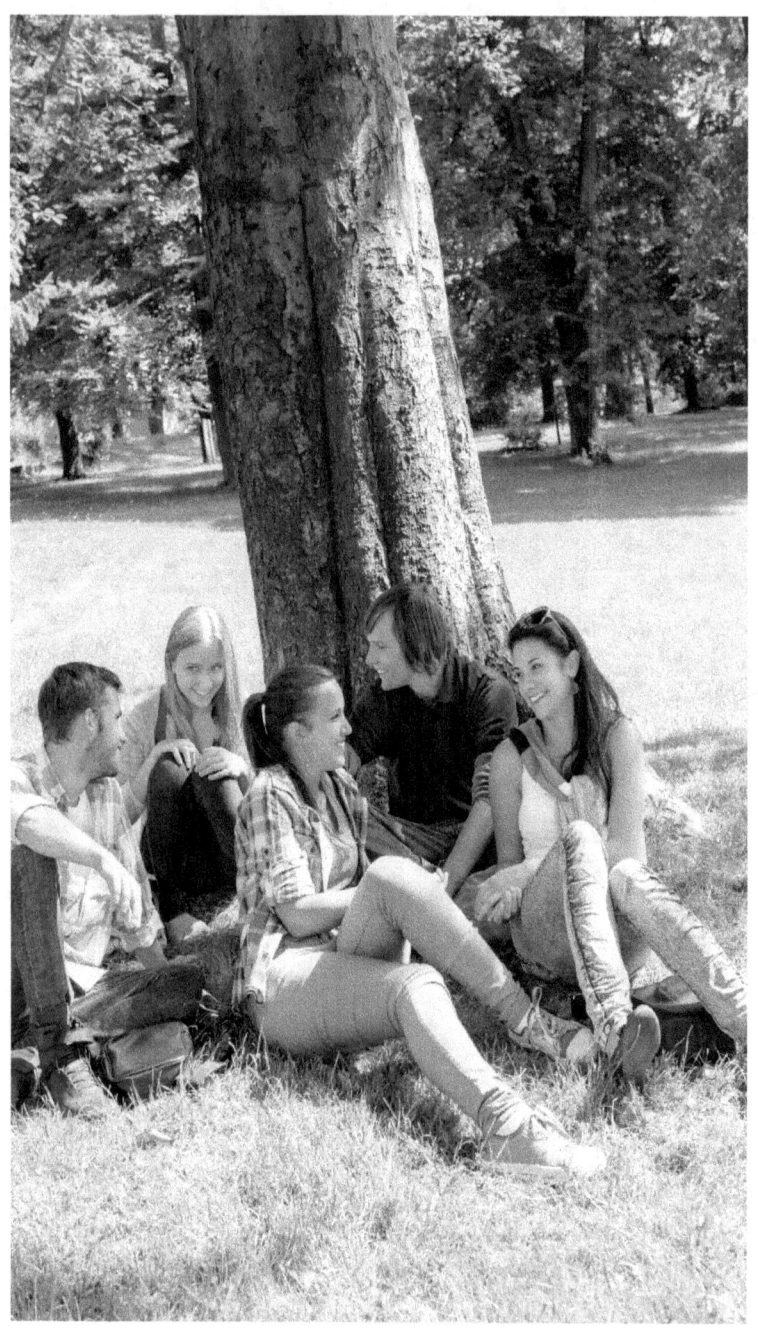

47. Maintain a Healthy Weight

There is a clear link between memory loss and obesity. Overweight individuals, upon examination, have been found to have less brain tissues and their brains seem years older compared to the brains of individuals with healthy weight. If you are overweight, you are likely to have more brain shrinkage that corresponds with loss of brain function.

It is therefore very important that you maintain your weight.

48. Stop Smoking

A single cigarette puff can reel in countless free radicals, which are oxygen molecules (unattached) that fight and kill brain cells. The action of these free radicals is similar to the way that oxygen causes rust on a metal.

Smoking can also increase the risk of developing Alzheimer's disease. Thus, quitting smoking is not a choice. Do it and have better brain health.

49. Limit Electromagnetic Field Exposure

An EMF (electromagnetic field) is created every time an electric current passes through a wire. Living in a world surrounded by EMFs is harmful to our brains in so many ways. They disrupt brain metabolism and production of neurotransmitters. They make brain cells leaky. They increase the risk of dementia and slow down reaction times.

The frequent use of mobile phones is in the same cancer-causing category as chloroform, engine exhaust, and lead. Plus, mobile phones are held directly to your brain, which makes them especially harmful. If you must use your phone all the time, get an EMF-filtering mobile phone case.

50. Get Adequate Sleep

Getting around 8 hours of sleep is crucial for your mental well-being and physical health. It is not an option. During sleep, the brain expels toxic debris, repairs itself, and collates memories. The lack of a good night's sleep will impair your attention, judgment, creativity, and memory.

A particular culprit is using electronics at night. They emit blue light that tells your brain that it is daytime, and not your time to sleep.

51. Limit Prescription Medication

Prescription medication can cause memory loss. Two of the worst culprits are prescription sleeping pills and statins to lower cholesterol. Consult your doctor about changing medications or, if possible, lowering the dose.

Chapter 6: 7 Powerful Natural Ways to Improve Brain Power in Kids Between 0-3 Years

Now that we have established fifty-one proven ones to boost your own brain power, we will delve into ways to enhance the brain power of your children as well- starting from the time they are born and moving forward from there. This chapter will address the importance of developing an early foundation to ensure better brain performance throughout your child's life. Giving your infant the greatest start in life mentally will enable them to master many things, including language, coordination, and other skills well before their peers. As we progress through this chapter we will discover seven different ways to ensure your infant or toddler can have the most optimal mental beginning that you can offer to him or her.

1. Start improving your child's brain power before he or she is even born.

Making healthy decisions throughout your pregnancy is a surefire way to set your baby up for success later in life. Many of the guidelines outlined earlier for boosting your own brain power are even more important to follow during pregnancy, and there are additional rules that you should keep in mind in order to provide your child with the best start possible. For instance, studies have shown that smoking during pregnancy can impact test scores of your child- for years or decades to come. As such, be sure you cut out such a harmful habit (and it will be better for your own health, too!). It may sound like a given, but any drug use should be avoided while gestating as well.

You may have heard that it is okay to have a glass of wine a day in pregnancy- but research suggests that drinking will have to go, too, if you desire optimal mental functioning for your son or daughter. Fetal alcohol syndrome disorder, or FASD, can occur from even small amounts of alcohol intake, and can result in damage to the brain and the central nervous system. This can result in microcephaly (a smaller than average head), which in some cases can also suggest reduced brain power. Additionally, it can cause impaired motor skills, learning disabilities, and much poorer than average scores when your child takes standardized tests later in life. While the scientific community is still not certain exactly how much alcohol is too much, if you want to enable your child to have the highest odds of being mentally successful, recommendations suggest that complete restraint will be your safest bet.

Finally, diet and exercise (especially the foods and activities suggested in chapter 5!), will ensure the healthiest possible offspring. Most of the recommended vitamins and nutrients can be achieved via daily use of a prenatal vitamin, but consult with your doctor to ensure you are successfully getting them all- for the good of both yourself and your future child.

2. Use physical touch often and strive to be attentive.

Especially when your child is very young, the importance of physical interaction cannot be overstated. Cuddles, caresses, and infant massage have all been shown to relax and focus infants and increase their overall health. So important is physical touch that an absence of regular tactile stimulation with another human being has been linked to a decreased brain size, as well as a greater likelihood of severe social and bonding problems that can persist throughout your child's life. Additionally, skin to skin contact with infants has been shown aid in a baby's ability to recognize itself and speeds up mental development. This is likely due to decreasing their stress levels, fostering a calm and pleasant environment for learning.

Besides accelerating mental expansion, attentiveness and physical contact show babies that their actions can have a real impact on the world and the people around them. Seeing a pattern of predictable responses to their actions- being held when they cry, laughing when they laugh, handing them things when they reach for them- demonstrates to even the youngest of children that what they do matters, and helps them to learn about patterns and what actions lead to what responses. Differences in infant responsiveness based on how their parents react to them can be seen as early as four months old, and possibly sooner- so it is important to give them a strong foundation from day one.

3. Talk to your baby or toddler- even before they can really talk back.

Babies and toddlers learn so quickly, and one of the things they master at phenomenal speeds is language. The more you talk to your infant the faster he or she will learn to speak as well. The "baby talk" method of speaking that many parents employ automatically can even be beneficial, as it frequently relies on drawing out syllables and sounds, enabling your child to better learn to vocalize the words they are hearing. When you diaper, feed, or play with your little one, talk to them about what you are doing. This will help them to understand words even before they can begin to say them themselves. Reading to your child from an early age can also be hugely beneficial here- and when they are a beginning to vocalize some words, you can even expand that to read with them as they remember more and more of their favorite stories. Finally, if you followed the earlier advice given in chapter five on learning a second language, speak and read to your child in that language as well. This will enable your offspring to grow up bilingual, which provides a significant mental step up for them throughout their life.

4. Sing to, and eventually with, your young child.

This might feel silly sometimes, but it has been done by parents in the form of lullabies for centuries, if not more. As your little one progresses into the toddler years, it will become even more important. The fun, interactive tunes for children are not just there to entertain them- they are valuable brain boosting opportunities. In addition to furthering language and communication skills (especially if you enjoy songs in multiple languages), many of these juvenile tunes involve dances or other motions in time to the music or words. Going through those together will increase your child's sense of rhythm. Lastly, singing songs will enhance your child's memory, as many people can remember songs and rhymes better than words alone.

5. Ensure adequate exposure to a variety of sensory activities.

This one might seem unpleasant to you as an adult at first, but it can be of great benefit to your child. By sensory play, we are referring to various materials with diverse textures- many of them will be messy, though! Letting your child play in sand and mud teaches them about the different properties of mixtures and allows them to understand the world around them better. This is accomplished naturally in many different ways- petting a dog, feeding themselves diverse finger foods, taking a bath, wearing clothing of differing fabric types- but it can be truly beneficial to help foster it as well.

Let your toddler touch items in nature, and describe to them what they are feeling. When they are old enough, ask them what it feels like to build their word skills. Some museums have sections enabling children to touch various more unusual objects- opportunities such as that should be seized when possible. By learning about a variety of shapes and compositions you teach your child how the world fits together and foster an early understanding of basic physics.

6. Enable your toddler to explore independently.

Of course, safety comes first, and supervision is important, but allowing your little one to traverse the world around them grants them a tremendous amount of early spatial awareness. Letting them crawl beneath things, climb on and over items, run far away and return to where he or she started are all invaluable to teaching your son or daughter about navigation and distance. This type of exploration also aids in motor control and an early learning of variance in geographical terrain. An easy and ideal place for such early learning can be found in most parks and playgrounds, which provide many child friendly features to play with and explore. Even a minor fall can help your child to better understand risk versus reward and to weigh consequences that their actions might have. If you are uncomfortable granting your little one too much independence outside the house, your own yard or home can still prove effective in helping them to learn these valuable mental skills.

7. Encourage and allow your child to help you.

At this stage of life, your toddler is likely watching and imitating everything that you do. Even though it is sometimes likely to be less than helpful, actively engaging your child in many of the activities they observe you doing can be very helpful, in particular clean up time. Categorizing toys and other things by type enables them to see patterns more clearly. Stacking books or other similar items allows them to determine cause and effect based on the size of which one goes on top to avoid the stack falling. Activities like stirring food while cooking can engage the senses and foster a further understanding of working for and waiting for rewards when they reap the benefits later. Even things like feeding and dressing themselves can teach them a lot about motor control and various materials. Whenever you have the time, fostering independence and allowing your child to help you is proven to enhance brain power and speed up learning.

Chapter 7: 7 Powerful Natural Ways to Improve Brain Power in Kids Between 4-8 Years

Has your child moves out of their toddler years, in which they were completely reliant on their parents, and into their school years, you will no doubt notice an increase in independence and in abilities, both physically and mentally. This is the stage of life in which a child begins to know more of who they are and starts to form their own friendships and activities, but they are still heavily attached and dependent on their parents for most things in life. They are capable of learning and doing more without your direct guidance, but are still open to what you have to say and are still closely watching what you do. In this chapter we will establish seven different ways to foster brain development in your school age child.

1. Play with your child.

At this stage of life your son or daughter is likely becoming more capable and willing to play without you, but they also still crave your attention. When the opportunity presents itself, join in on your child's games. Play the character that they want you to play or get on the ground with them and take part in their lego building or barbie games. Solicit their ideas, though- don't provide too many yourself. This fosters their creativity and shows them that their thoughts and words lead to actions. Additionally, playing with them helps them to build social skills and facilitates bonding. Finally, consider having a family board game night. This allows you to spend time with them and develop their social skills while also encouraging them to think about strategy and aiding them in enhancing their foresight.

2. Encourage imaginative play.

This builds on the previous point and should definitely be engaged in while playing with your child, but can be just as effective or even more so when done alone or with other children. Pretending to be characters from books, films, or televisions, with special powers or unusual circumstances, enables your child to put themselves into someone else's shoes to an extent. It also inspires them to come up with 'plots' for their own stories. The characters they are playing as need a mission or a goal, after all. Creating story lines can greatly enhance brain power, especially if they must solve problems or overcome adversities in their make believe games. This same concept can apply when playing with dolls or action figures as well, as your child determines what the characters think or feel and how they will respond to their circumstances. Other creative games such as building blocks (especially the type without a kit or clear goal) can really stimulate a growing mind and encourage it to formulate its own story line and its own solutions, which are guaranteed ways to increase brain power.

3. Provide certain foods.

Much like adults, children can also benefit greatly from consuming or not consuming certain foods and from ensuring certain nutritional needs are adequately and appropriately met. Most of the guidelines offered in chapter five for adult nutrition apply here as well and as such we shall not repeat them, but we will discuss a few items particularly recommended for children here.

We'll begin our discussion on childhood nutrition with a suggestion to consider feeding your child eggs. Scrambled, boiled, poached-however your son or daughter prefers them, they are a natural brain-boosting food highly recommended for your child. In addition to containing vitamin B12, which we established the benefits of in chapter 5, they are also high in protein, vitamin A, vitamin D, and vitamin E, all of which are very important for growing children. Perhaps more importantly, the egg yolks contain choline, which is proven to enhance memory, and iron, which is linked to optimal brain functioning.

Another important food to serve for your child is beans. Black beans, kidney beans, garbanzo beans- any type of bean will do, though kidney and pinto beans might be the most effective at boosting brain function. Beans are packed with omega 3 fatty acids, which encourages brain growth and increases brain functioning. Additionally, beans contain lots of fiber, which makes you feel fuller longer and increases energy. This can be invaluable for keeping your child focused on learning throughout the school day. Prepared in a burrito, as a side dish, as a major ingredient of a chili or in less traditional choices like hummus, beans can go a long way towards enhancing your child's mental faculties.

Lastly, you might want to consider offering your child cheese, either as a snack or on sandwiches. The fat content in cheese might deter some adults, but for a growing child it is just fine, and as we established, fat can boost the brain. Additionally, cheese is a nutritionally-dense food rich in calcium and vitamin D- a vitamin desperately needed by children, who need up to ten times more than the recommended adult serving. This can enhance the neurological system and boost brain power and coordination.

4. Establish a homework routine.

Developing a regular schedule to complete homework can ensure that your child is prepared and in the right mindset each day when it comes time to attend to their studies. Set and maintain a consistent time that homework must be dealt with, and strive to limit exceptions to the rule. In an ideal world, ensure it is still during daytime hours, as natural circadian rhythms will cause your child to be more alert and focused before the sun sets. It is also exceedingly helpful to ensure that the same room and setting are selected each time, as this causes people to be conditioned to view that environment as a place to learn. You may even want to consider aromatherapy. A number of different herbal choices have been shown to be effective in improving memory and concentration, in particular rosemary and peppermint. Employing essential oils in the room your child will study in can increase their focus and ability to learn, as well as teaching them to link those scents to getting their schoolwork done, which will serve as a built in mood adjustment tool. Routine is very important for young children and following these guidelines will certify that their study time is effective.

5. Teach your children ways to calm down.

Stress can happen at any age, and when it does, it makes learning and mental tasks much more difficult. Many children are not yet aware of coping techniques or of healthy and effective ways to deal with their anxiety when it occurs. First off, talk to them frankly about stress and worry and let them know that it is normal and can be handled productively. Then, we can take inspiration from the meditation tips for adults found in chapter five- but in a more simplified, child friendly format. Envisioning a calm, pleasant, peaceful activity can help a child develop a sense of calm. Have them breathe out while imagining blowing on a dandelion or a birthday candle, and breathe in as though they are smelling freshly baked cookies. You can also instruct them in deep breathing techniques, where the air moves up through their bodies and out. Present it in a fun, simplified way, and remind your child to employ it when they feel anxious and need to calm down. It can become a nice, focusing habit that enables greater concentration and enhanced cerebral functioning.

6. Stick to one task at a time.

For adults, we discussed the benefits of limiting how often you multitask. This is even more important for children, which is why we revisit it here. Children can easily be overstimulated by too much input, especially of the visual variety. Cut off television, music, and other sources of distraction when they are studying or working on a hobby. Provide regular breaks to ensure they do not become overloaded and unable to focus, but during study time or structured play time, ensure they are not distracted by anything. It has been shown to greatly reduce the effectiveness of the developing brain when it is forced to multitask, and is certainly not worth any slight increase in work efficiency.

7. Ask open ended questions often.

You are no doubt aware that children are naturally inquisitive and are therefore constantly asking questions. This innate curiosity builds the mental faculties and should be encouraged- but not simply by answering their questions. If your child asks you a question, do your best to turn it around on them. Ask them why they think it is like that, and really try to urge them to consider the possibilities. Once they answer, keep the discussion going for as long as you can, conversing back and forth about the possible reasons for their every question. Eventually, you can tell them the answer, of course- but it would be even better to enable them to look it up, online or in a book, and learn for themselves after considering all different choices. This method of discussion really enhances critical thinking and problem solving skills and teaches children to truly think for themselves, which is an invaluable ability to have throughout their lives.

Chapter 8: 7 Powerful Natural Ways to Improve Brain Power in Kids Between 9-14 Years

The ages between 9-14 can be fraught with changes. It is the stage where puberty usually begins and is commonly the beginnings of truly exercising independence. Children at this age are trying to figure out who they are, what they like, and what they plan to become. Generally, they are less dependent on their parents at this age, but that does not mean they are not amenable to strategies and tips to improve their brain power and functioning in what is still crucial developmental years. Here we will discuss seven excellent methods of fostering brain growth and function as your child enters his or her teen years.

1. Make a designated time or activity to talk and connect with your child.

This is a continuation of the open ended questions that we recommended employing with younger children. You can still do that, but at your children get older it might become more theoretical or philosophical. This enables both of you to consider aspects and perspectives you might otherwise not have thought of. It also allows you to be a continued influential presence as your child gets older and to remain connected in their life, and what better way to accomplish that than a strategy that also boosts their growing brain? In order to encourage your son or daughter to open up to you a bit, it helps to have an environment in which you are used to sharing thoughts and events with each other. One easy option is a scheduled family dinner each night, full of food and conversation. If you'd rather something more private, a fun evening once a week with just you and your child can work wonders here.

2. Encourage them to learn to play a musical instrument.

This is an age in which children are frequently becoming more interested in music. While many of us are less than fond of the musical tastes of our tweens, it can be an excellent way to encourage them to learn to play a musical instrument. Talk to them about what options might appeal to them and consider getting them an instrument and lessons. Studies have shown that musical training has significant brain boosting abilities in children and in teens, and also aids in lowering anxiety, enabling them to learn more effectively. It doesn't just enhance their sense of rhythm- it actually has been shown to improve scientific and mathematical comprehension and raises standardized test scores overall. Research even suggests that IQ can experience an average of a three-point rise from studying music- a worthy investment for a growing brain.

3. Make sure they are eating a healthy breakfast.

You know the common saying that 'breakfast is the most important meal of the day'? That could be debated for adults, but for children and teens, research suggests that it rings true. A nutritious breakfast, ideally full of fiber, ensures that children are alert, energized, and ready to learn- and keeps them feeling that way until they near lunchtime and can replenish. In addition to being more focused, a daily breakfast has been shown to foster memory growth and improvement- because all that learning in class does little good if they forget it by the time they get home. Strive to avoid sweet treats in the morning, and make sure to not let them skip breakfast entirely. Their developing brains truly benefit from the early morning energy source.

4. Encourage periodic use of their non-dominant hand.

This one is a little bit strange, but it can be an interesting and fun challenge for children in this age range. Doing so engages and stimulates the brain and new and unexpected ways, allowing for increased growth. We touched briefly on brain lateralization- the concept that the right brain controls the left side of the body and vice versa- way back in chapter two, and it comes into play here. The side of the body you don't use as extensively is not just causing you physical ineptness- your brain is clumsier on that side when it comes to motions as well. Additionally, the right brain is commonly considered more creative, while the left is considered more analytical. Want to boost your skills in one of those areas? Use the hand for it. Try to make it a fun game or goal for your children, and watch their brain power blossom.

5. Ensure that they experience some boredom or down time.

When we speak of down time here, what we mean is complete down time. No computer, no tablet, no smart phone or television. Just time in which your child has to occasionally be alone with their thoughts. Ideally, this time should be spent outdoors, as with a bit of creativity it is easy to find ways to entertain yourself out of doors, and the benefits of spending time in nature apply to children as well as adults. In our modern day world, we are constantly searching for something to entertain us, usually something electronic. Rarely do we stop to think about what we want to do, what we can do- but it is very important to do so to boost our brain power and our creativity. Allow them to do what they like- but do not provide them with snacks or entertainment, and deny them their electronics during this time period. It does not have to occur often or complaints might grow too strong, but perhaps once or twice a week could be a time to unplug. This will force your teen to entertain themselves for a change instead of simply being entertained, and in doing so, they will exercise their brains.

6. Motivate them to discover their passion- or at least to adopt a hobby.

One of the easy ways to foster such motivation is to follow the previous recommendation here. It will really inspire your child to come up with activities that interest them. When they do, consider signing them up for classes or providing them with the necessary equipment so they can practice something they might come to love. At this stage of life, children are figuring out who they are and what they want to do with their lives. Being able to test the waters and truly engage in a passion of theirs is wonderful in developing their sense of self. Almost any skill they might want to learn- dance, sports, art, etc- will endow your child with enhanced critical thinking creative skills. Every time they practice their hobby, they are exercising their brains, efficiently boosting their brain power and cognitive functions.

7. Incite them to spend time in self-reflection.

At this age in life children are going through a lot of changes. They are pulling away from their parents and learning about who they are and what they want. It is the start of a more independent and also more rebellious era. They might feel anxious, worried, and stressed more often than they used to as they go through these changes, and it is likely they will not be as comfortable just leaning on you as they once were. Impulse control can frequently be a problem here, which can lead them down risky paths. To help counter this, urge your child to spend time getting to know who they are. Online quizzes and tests can make this fun, as can books, discussion, and other tools. Help them to understand that their desires and whims are normal, as are their mood swings-but teach them to, whenever they want to act on something, to pause and consider the effects of their actions. Groom them to automatically weigh the risks and the rewards, and then to consider if the end results will truly suit what they want as a person. This will help them to learn about long term planning, cause and effect, and responsibility. The ability to think ahead effectively is an important life-long skill that the brain should grow used to exercising early in life.

Conclusion

Take Care of Your Brain

As you can see from the 72 methods mentioned in this book, taking care of the brain is not just about solving riddles and engaging in crossword puzzles. It is also about changing your lifestyle. Fortunately, most of the changes are so simple that they can be applied right away.

Follow these 72 methods and see how they guide you to develop a better memory which will make you feel happier, more focused, and more fulfilled in life.

Thank you for reading this book.

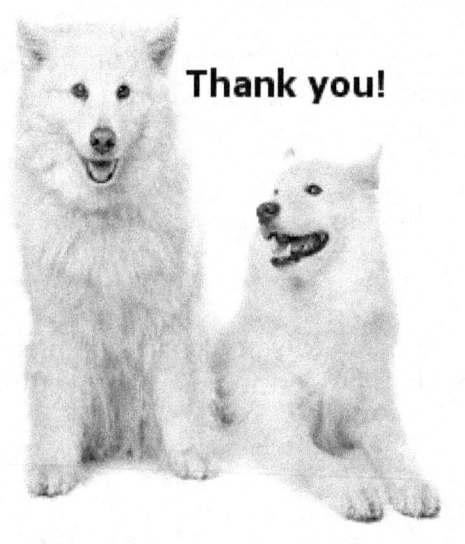

Thank you!

We really hope it has helped you in understanding the brain and how its power can be enhanced significantly.

Can we now ask you for a small favor?

We would like to take this book to as many people as possible and help them too in realizing the full potential of their brain thus enabling them to lead better lives.

Please help us in this effort.

If you liked this book, can you please recommend it and post your feedback.

Please go to the review page **http://amzn.to/1QrhdOe** and post your thoughts.

As a thank you for reading our book and for posting your review, we would like to give you some BONUS GIFTS.

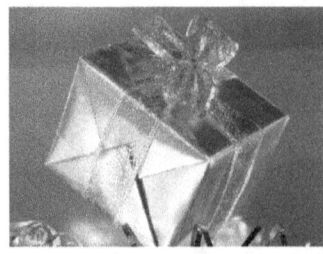

Get Your BONUS!

A Beginners Guide to Demystifying Meditation and Being Mindful

A must read book for everyone. This is what you will learn in this book -

- The Development & Origins Of Meditation

- Benefits Of Meditating Daily

- Different Techniques Of Meditation

- Relaxation & Mindfulness Uncovered

- The Sub Conscious, Dreams & Meditation

- Healing Emotional Wounds

Please go to our website www.shininguniverseenergy.com to download.

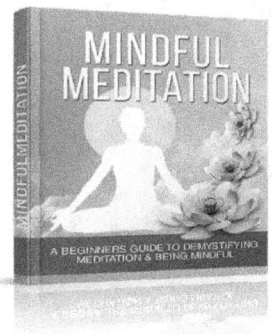

The Power of Goals

Learn How to Set Goals in Life, How to Stick to Your Goals and Achieve Them.

Get This Book and Accomplish More in Life!

Please go to our website www.shininguniverseenergy.com to download

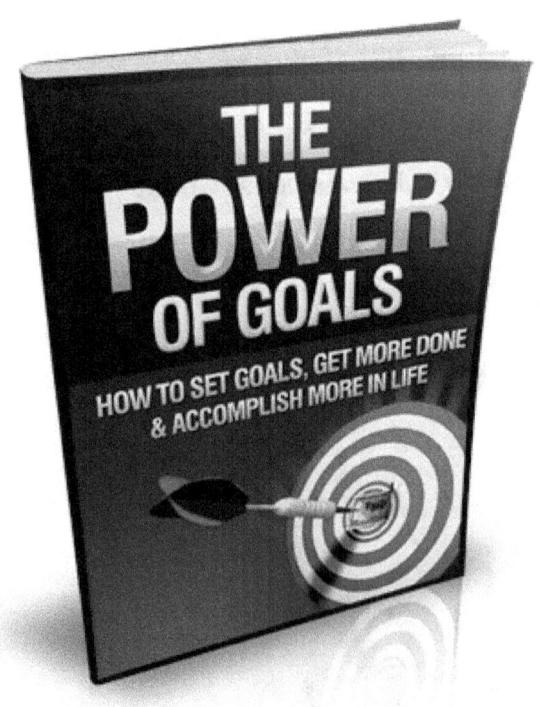

What is Time Management – Your Basic Guide to Understanding Time Management

Get this fabulous book and learn the below –

- The Basics on Time Management

- The Basics on Project Management

- The Basics on Personal Knowledge Management

- Creating an Effective Environment

- Setting Priorities Basics and Goals Basics

- Implementing Goals Basics

  Please go to our website www.shininguniverseenergy.com to download.

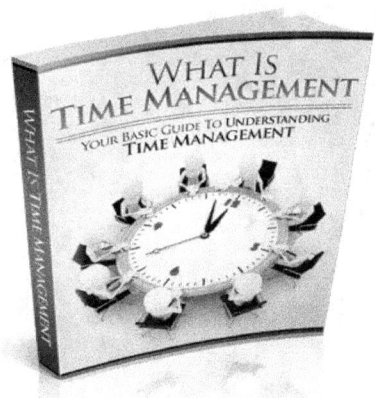

Breaking the Habits of Sexual Addictions

Learn how to live clean and regain your self-respect. This book will tell you –

- When Is Sex Actually an Addiction

- Myths

- Getting on the Road to Recovery

- Means to Recovery

- Changes to Make

Please go to our website
www.shininguniverseenergy.com to download.

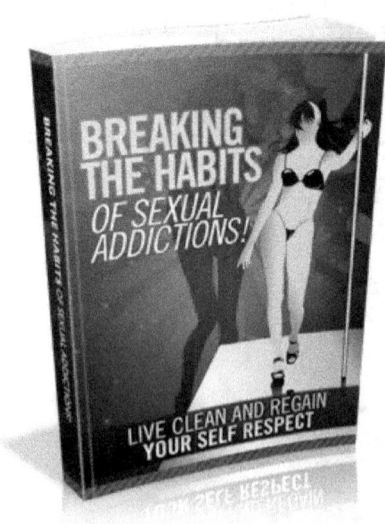

50 Tips to Boost Your Productivity

You need this book to learn how to do more with less.

The tips mentioned in this book are a must read for everyone – whether you are a Student, a Professional or a Business-man.

Please go to our website www.shininguniverseenergy.com to download.

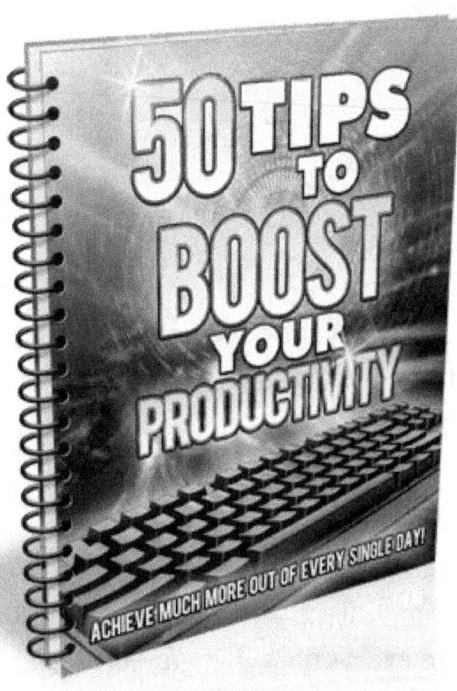

We hope you liked your bonus gifts.

Please do visit us on our website
www.ShiningUniverseEnergy.com

We would love to see you there!

Like us on Facebook
https://www.facebook.com/ShiningUniversEe
nergy

Follow us on Twitter @ShiningUE

'Shining Universe Energy' is a platform for spreading love, light and happiness to all.

Through our publishing unit **'Shining Universe Energy Books'** we aim to bring out books that will enrich lives, inspire and motivate everyone to become bigger and better.

Our efforts are also aimed at trying to cultivate positive thinking and to make our society a better place to live.

We really hope our books will enable readers to solve their problems and help them lead meaningful lives.

Do you want to know about our other book?

Please see the information on the next page.

Invite happiness into your life by learning 101 powerful NATURAL techniques and be free of depression, stress and anxiety forever. This book is for everyone who want to lead a happier and healthier life.

'Depression: 101 Powerful Ways to Beat Depression, Stress, Anxiety and Be Happy NATURALLY!

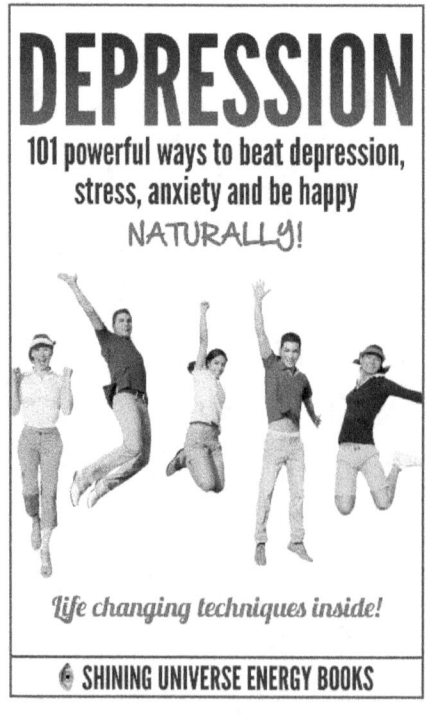

You can buy it right now on Amazon –

USA readers – Please go to
http://amzn.to/1XIOrvD

UK readers - Please go to
http://amzn.to/1RV7ZYx

Readers from all other countries can get the book here **lrd.to/Depression**

This book is also available in bookstores worldwide.

You can order a print-on-demand copy too. Please go to the below address -
https://www.createspace.com/5939934

Thank you and good luck!

www.ingramcontent.com/pod-product-compliance
Lightning Source LLC
Chambersburg PA
CBHW071819200526
45169CB00018B/444